Heike Steinhoff (ed.)
Epidemics and Othering

## Editorial

Since national histories have been discredited as the only legitimate way to write history, global history has been gaining momentum. Global history, however, is not merely "history outside Europe"; and global is more than "around the world". Global history means historiography that tries to overcome Eurocentric perspectives and to focus on global complexity and interrelations. Thus, global historians tend to study topics such as colonialism, migration, trade, international cooperation, slavery, tourism, imperialism, globalization, knowledge transfers, etc.

The book series **Global and Colonial History** offers a common forum to discuss cutting-edge research on these issues. We consider colonial and imperial history to be a central part of global history because it is exemplary of this historiography as a history of interrelations and because it challenges past and present power structures and hegemonic discourses on a methodological level.

**Heike Steinhoff** is Junior Professor of American Studies at Ruhr-Universität Bochum. Her research focuses on American media culture from the 19th to the 21st century, gender studies, body studies, and urban studies. She is the author of two monographs, one on makeovers and monstrosities in American culture and the other one on pirates in Hollywood cinema. She has also published on hipster culture, literary discourses of urban sexuality in 19th century America, gender in children's movies, filmic representations of metropolitan masculinities, and the interrelations of body positivity, self-help literature and popular feminisms.

Heike Steinhoff (ed.)

# Epidemics and Othering

The Biopolitics of COVID-19
in Historical and Cultural Perspectives

[transcript]

**Bibliographic information published by the Deutsche Nationalbibliothek**
The Deutsche Nationalbibliothek lists this publication in the Deutsche Nationalbibliografie; detailed bibliographic data are available in the Internet at http://dnb.d-nb.de

© 2024 transcript Verlag, Bielefeld

Cover layout: Kordula Röckenhaus, Bielefeld
Cover illustration: Pete Linforth on Pixabay

https://doi.org/10.14361/9783839465059
Print-ISBN: 978-3-8376-6505-5
PDF-ISBN: 978-3-8394-6505-9
ISSN of series: 2701-0309
eISSN of series: 2702-9328

# Contents

# List of Figures

# Acknowledgments

This book has its roots in an international digital symposium at Ruhr University Bochum, Germany, organized together with my colleague Rebecca Brückmann at the height of the COVID-19 pandemic in 2021. Our great collaboration not only contributed to a successful symposium, but also shaped the first outline of this book. Many thanks to all contributors to this volume, some of whom were part of the initial symposium and some of whom joined this project at a later stage. I also want to thank the team at transcript for their support, particularly Mirjam Galley, whose immediate interest in this project paved the way for its publication. Finally, I would like to acknowledge the excellent work and commitment of my research assistant, Claudia Eugenie Laube. This book could not have been completed without her invaluable support in formatting, proofreading and organizing all stages of the preparation of the manuscript.

# 1. Biopolitics, Othering, and the COVID-19 Pandemic: A Critical Introduction

*Heike Steinhoff*

In autumn 2021, at the height of the global coronavirus pandemic, a digital international symposium at Ruhr University Bochum, Germany, explored the historical, cultural, and narrative frames that shaped discourses on the contemporary pandemic in different (trans)national and glocal contexts. The particular focus of the symposium that sparked the idea to this book was the historical and cultural significance of the pandemic and what my colleague and co-organizer, Rebecca Brückmann, and I then called the biopolitics of COVID-19.[1] Like many scholars that have explored the biopolitics of the pandemic over the past three years, we took our concept of biopolitics from Michel Foucault. In his work, the term is somewhat elusive but mainly functions to describe a distinct technology of power directed at the regulation of life and populations. Biopolitics emerged at the end of the eighteenth century and was linked to the rise of European liberalism. It "focused on the species body, the body imbued with the mechanics of life and serving as the basis of the biological processes: propagation, births and mortality, the level of health, life expectancy and longevity, with all the conditions that can cause these to vary" (Foucault [1978] 1990, 139). According to Foucault, "[t]heir supervision was effected through an entire series of interventions and *regulatory controls: a biopolitics of the population*" ([1978] 1990, 139). By replacing the "ancient right to *take* life or *let* live," associated with sovereign power, biopower is "a power to *foster* life or *disallow* it to the point of death" ([1978] 1990, 138). These concepts of biopolitics and biopower, as I am going to discuss in this introduction,

---

1    This introduction is in parts based on our welcome address to this symposium, jointly written and presented by Brückmann and Steinhoff in October 2021. Many thanks to Kornelia Freitag and Chris Katzenberg for their invaluable feedback on a first draft of the introduction to this volume.

resonated with the measures and modes of governmentality implemented by many countries around the globe during the COVID-19 pandemic.

The second, and closely linked historical-cultural process that had sparked our interest and led to the symposium and this book, is the one of 'othering,' the discursive marking of bodies and groups of people that are seen as different from the self. While the construction of an 'other' might be central to identity formation and constitutive of the notion of 'a self,' the concept of othering describes processes of stigmatization, marginalization, exclusion, and subordination in a context of hierarchical, hegemonic power relations (e.g. Spivak 1985). For most of humanity's history, epidemics and pandemics have been shaped by the idea of contagion as an invisible foe, supposedly hidden in dirty surroundings or substances, dirty air, miasmas, and other(ed) people. Up to today epidemiology has developed into an empirical and statistical science that studies the microorganisms and processes responsible for the spread of infectious diseases. Yet, a cultural-historical approach shows that in the contemporary COVID-19 pandemic, the need to 'make sense' of a senseless epidemic mobilized long-established tropes of cultural othering just as in previous epidemics and pandemics. In the current age of globalization, which has also been referred to as an "age of universal contagion" (Hardt and Negri 2001, 136), the politics of othering are closely linked with biopolitics in myriad forms. The intertwinement of these politics with their specific historical, geographic, and cultural shapes, functions, and effects is the focus that unites the multi- and interdisciplinary contributions collected in this book. In this introduction, I will sketch the frame for these case studies by illuminating some of the entanglements of biopolitics and othering in the context of the COVID-19 pandemic.

## COVID-19 and Biopolitics

Caused by a novel virus, SARS-CoV-2 (severe acute respiratory syndrome coronavirus 2), the coronavirus disease 19 (COVID-19) was first identified in Wuhan, China, in December 2019. Soon, it spread worldwide, with the World Health Organization declaring COVID-19 a Public Health Emergency of International Concern in January 2020 (2020a), and calling it a pandemic in March 2020 (2020b). As of April 3, 2023, more than 760 million cases and 6,88 million deaths due to the virus have been reported globally (World Health Organization 2023). Governments and institutions around the world have implemented various and sometimes divergent measures in their attempts to stop the virus, 'flatten the curve,' prevent overburdens of hospital capacities, facilitate research for a vaccine, purchase and distribute vaccinations when a vaccine was found, and 'care' for their populations. Accordingly, many scholars have since used the concept of biopolitics to explore the politics behind measures, such as the restrictions on movement in forms of lockdowns, quarantines, or closed borders, the management of medical treatments, the employment of tracking and surveillance technologies, and different forms of recommendations or reinforcements of vaccination, as well as to analyze the (in)discriminate patterns of the spread of the virus in different spaces and communities. Already in 2020, when the concept of biopolitics became increasingly mobilized in academic and also public discussions, Philipp Sarasin remarked: "It looks like a biopolitical dream: governments, advised by physicians, impose pandemic dictatorship on entire populations. Getting rid of all democratic obstacles under the pretext of 'health,' even 'survival,' they are finally able to govern the population as they have, more or less openly, always done in modernity: as pure 'biomass'" (2020).

However, Sarasin warns of such an application of the term biopolitics, as the notion of a "dictatorship" of biopolitics can be misleading.[2] In fact, Foucault has emphasized time and again that power is not something one holds but is both repressive and subjective, "intentional and nonsubjective," no superstructure, but intrinsic to relations, "the name that one attributes to a complex strategical situation in a particular society" ([1978] 1990, 93; 92–7). Hence, biopolitics needs to be understood as a highly complex process and as taking historically, geographically, and culturally different forms. Accordingly, as Daniele Lorenzini suggests, this also means that "it would be wise for us to refuse the 'blackmail' of biopolitics: we do not have to be 'for' or 'against' it, … but address it as a historical event that still defines, at least in part, the way in which we are governed, the way in which we think about politics and about ourselves" (2021, S41). Also, Maurizio Meloni has called for a historicized perspective on biopolitics (2022), in his critique of Giorgio "Agamben's denunciation of COVID-19 as just another form of the state of exception that has lent power to experts who illegitimately occupy or monopolize the fuller philosophical sense of life" (60). Agamben's rejection and criticism of the political measures implemented in democratic nations to prevent a further spread of the

---

2    Sarasin suggests that three models described by Foucault as different forms of government in the context of three infectious diseases, leprosy, plague, and smallpox, might be more helpful in capturing the reality of government during the pandemic (2020).

virus as mechanisms of totalitarian control have been highly controversial, in Meloni's words: "Agamben's case very much reflects the limitation of a certain social constructionist and ultimately idealistic understanding of the biological importance of health and the tragedy of disembodied speculation" (60).[3] Also Lorenzini has suggested that "if we just insist on coercive measures, on being confined, controlled, and 'trapped' at home during these *extraordinary* times, we risk overlooking the fact that disciplinary and biopolitical power mainly functions in an automatic, invisible, and perfectly *ordinary* way—and that it is most dangerous precisely when we do not notice it" (2021, S42). Thus, while the ways in which biopower and specific biopolitics are at work might be especially visible during times of crisis or a declared state of emergency, such as the COVID-19 pandemic, these times are not exceptional in making us biopolitical subjects.[4]

If anything, the past years with the Corona pandemic seem to have highlighted and accelerated societal developments and political trends. These include, but are in no ways limited to, the medicalization of all facets of life (with the side-effect that many people seem to feel to have become medical experts on viruses, aerosols, and vaccines), the politicization of medicine,[5] and the 'statisticization' of society, as mortality rates and other corona-related statistics have been displayed in the media on a daily basis. Moreover, around the world, but particularly in the Global North, we have seen rapid digitalization (most contributors to this volume have never met each other in person but have instead become experienced in online teaching and digital conferences, such as the one that turned into this volume). Thus, long-lasting discussions about the digital divide and media competence have gained new urgency. Some positive effects of lockdowns on the natural environment and the notion of the global pandemic's relation to the ignorance of ecological transformations in the context of climate change, have shaped responses to the ecological and planetary dimensions of the contemporary disease. Lockdowns, quarantines, masks, and tracking technologies have become the focal point of debates regarding governmental power and governmentality,

---

3    Cf. also Tim Christiaens (2021) for a detailed analysis of Giorgio Agamben's public interventions in the context of the COVID-19 pandemic.

4    Cf. e.g. also Schubert (2020, 2022) and others on the notion that this is not a state of exception.

5    Cf. also Esposito in an interview with Tim Christiaens and Stijn De Cauwer (2020).

discussing civil liberties, and conceptualizing individual and collective freedoms in juxtaposition to discourses and measures of security, surveillance, and mobilities. The pandemic has heightened ethnic nationalist panics about migration, has increased anti-Asian violence, and has affected marginalized communities, particularly People of Color, significantly harder across the globe, both in terms of economic depravations, illness and mortality, and in terms of racism and anti-Semitism (cf. e.g. Navarro and Hernandez 2022). At the same time, amidst the coronavirus pandemic, the BlackLivesMatter movement reached new heights of visibility and participation, with US-wide and international protests after George Floyd died as the result of a violent police arrest in May 2020. This is only a cursory, and necessarily limited list of some of the developments related to the contemporary pandemic, one that is shaped by the situatedness of my own knowledge (Haraway 1988) and experience of the pandemic.

## COVID-19 and the Politics of Othering

The COVID-19 pandemic and the biopolitical regulations that it sparked have affected all facets of life and its effects have been experienced both by collective and individual bodies in myriad different ways; ways that have been shaped by such factors as geographical location, nationality, age, dis/ability, gender, race, ethnicity, class, profession, etc. And like in previous epidemics and pandemics, it is this context that has produced and amplified processes of othering by COVID-19. The concept of othering, which originated in postcolonial (cf. e.g. Spivak 1985; Said 1978; Bhabha 1983) and feminist (cf. e.g. de Beauvoir [1948] 2010; hooks 1984; Hill Collins 1990; Butler 1993) theory, characterizes hegemonic processes of marking the differences between a supposedly superior 'We' and a supposedly inferior 'Other.' [6] Othering processes thus function to (re)produce social hierarchies and power relations by constructing marginalized groups as Other while simultaneously constructing the normative self. In particular in times of perceived social crisis, people tend to "resort to othering—dissociating themselves from the threat and blaming others—other

---

6    This volume follows the convention established in many works of postcolonial theory of using the spelling 'Other' with capital O. In contrast, Spivak, who builds upon the work of Jacques Lacan, differentiates between 'Other' (as Symbolic Other or imperial center) and 'other' (as the colonized, marginalized subjects).

countries, foreigners, stigmatized groups or other minorities, which helps reduce the powerlessness experienced during the crisis (Eichelberger, 2007)" (Li and Nicholson 2021). The emergence and spread of infectious diseases have occurred regularly throughout history, and major pandemics and epidemics such as the plague, cholera, typhoid, the flu, different variants of SARS, and MERS, have had significant impacts on humanity, often amplifying not only health but also sociocultural anxieties. Historically, this dynamic was intensified in times of increased mobility, which multiplies a perceived risk of contagion by the Other. According to historian Jim Downs, diseases emerged in the modern era "as crucial to imperialist adventures: By studying the spread of disease throughout the world, mapping its coordinates, pinpointing its origin, and defining its behavior, physicians developed key epidemiological methods" (2021, 35). The othering and subsequent racialization of Indigenous people, land, and spaces went hand in hand with these efforts. Historical research has demonstrated the close interrelations of colonialism, epidemics, and biopolitics, hence some scholars also challenge Foucault's argument that biopolitics emerged as the dominant mode of governmentality only at the end of the eighteenth century. As Carlos Jáuregui and David Solodkow argue in their study of Bartolomé de las Casas and sixteenth-century Spanish colonialism:

> Biopolitical analyses (of a Eurocentric Foucauldian cut) have generally ignored the specific experiences of domination and colonial government of life that followed the 'discovery' of America, when many human groups were seen, subjugated, and governed as human flocks: viz., submitted to processes of conversion; displaced from one area to another, from one continent to the next; racialized, reduced, and confined so as to be better governed and better exploited. (2018, 131–2) [7]

According to Jáuregui and Solodkow the "colonial designs for governing life and exploiting work were not 'precursors' to biopolitics; they were fully biopolitical" (2018, 132).

Sometimes, as a global pandemic the Corona virus has been perceived as 'a great leveler' of socioeconomic backgrounds and racialized identities. Yet,

---

7    The specific technologies, structures and agents of governmentality differed from the ones analyzed in Foucault's work in terms of historical and cultural/geographical context, in that they were not yet state centered and in that they were not only addressed at the body, but also at the spirit, in what the authors call "pneumo-politics" (2018, 129).

quite to the contrary, it has affected marginalized communities disproportionately. COVID-19 led to a rejuvenation and permutation of discourses that promote the othering of social groups also in states of (perceived) normalcy; often revealing the legacies of colonialism and other enduring structures of territorialization, discrimination, exploitation, and stigmatization. As Judith Butler wrote, already in March 2020:

> [T]he failure of some states or regions to prepare in advance (the US is now perhaps the most notorious member of that club), the bolstering of national policies and the closing of borders (often accompanied by panicked xenophobia), and the arrival of entrepreneurs eager to capitalize on global suffering, all testify to the rapidity with which radical inequality, nationalism, and capitalist exploitation find ways to reproduce and strengthen themselves within the pandemic zones.

Similarly, Lorenzini has argued that "biopolitics is always a politics of *differential vulnerability*. Far from being a politics that erases social and racial inequalities by reminding us of our common belonging to the same biological species, it is a politics that structurally relies on the establishment of hierarchies in the value of lives, producing and multiplying vulnerability as a means of governing people" (2021, S43–4).

This points to the intricate connection of biopolitics, as directed at the management of life and health, to what Achille Mbembe has called necropolitics, politics directed at the production of death and destruction (2003; 2019). As a critical lens, the notion of necropolitics enables us to shed light on the ways in which biopolitical policies 'let die': "Necropolitics ... uncovers how certain bodies are cultivated for life and (re)production while others are systemically marked for death, constructing a constantly shifting borderline between subjects deemed 'productive' and 'lawful' and non-subjects branded as 'illegitimate' or 'illegal'"(Quinan and Thiele 2020, 3). A differentiating look discloses that not all biopolitical measures implemented by different governmental or non-governmental institutions during the coronavirus pandemic have been the same. Esposito, for example, describes the strategy of natural 'herd immunity' followed by some countries at some points during the pandemic as an 'alternative' to the more widespread biopolitics of lockdowns, quarantines and later vaccinations, as "even thanatopolitical, because it entails the deaths of a considerable number of people who would otherwise live" (Christiaens and De Cauwer 2020). Vito Laterza and Louis Romer characterize the policy of 'herd immunity' as a form of "eugenics of the market" (2020). Similar arguments apply to those states that infamously and with severe consequences ignored or rejected the life-threatening reality of the virus, for example Brazil under President Jair Bolsonaro.[8] As Mark Howard argues,

> COVID-19, in making death visible, in bringing necropolitics into a field of visibility, has also made visible who in our own societies has been rendered expendable and who must necessarily be exposed to death: the elderly, the homeless, racial minorities, immigrants, rural populations; those who are unproductive or whose productivity is so essential that their lives can be given up to the priority of economic continuity. (2022, 2)

The geographies of infection and vulnerabilization[9] have revealed that 'health' is neither a universal nor clearly defined value (cf. Sparke and Anguelov 2020). Differential vulnerabilities could be witnessed in the different ways in which the pandemic affected communal and individual bodies based on their nation of origin, race, ethnicity, class, gender, sexualities, dis/abilities and other factors, often in ways that have reproduced hegemonic ideologies and modes of exclusions and othering. The COVID-19 pandemic has had, for instance, a disproportionate impact on women, for reasons such as gender-based differences in access to health care, gendered labor markets, domestic violence, and gendered expectations in terms of caregiving (cf. e.g. UN WOMEN 2020; Kupfer and Stutz 2022). Moreover, governmental regulations often privileged heteronormative families in their management of contact restrictions, for example in Germany during the Christmas period (Schubert 2020). Repeated outbreaks of the virus in the meat packing industry, among migrant workers, and in refugee camps revealed and exacerbated unjust working and living conditions, class differences and processes of marginalization based on ethnicity and national status (cf. also Schubert 2022). Repeatedly, in public discourses in many countries, the fear of the disease and the threat of its invisibility and uncontrollability, have been projected onto the social or cultural-ethnic Other, sparking othering processes along vectors of social differentiation, fostering

---

8    Cf. e.g. Cavalcanti Muniz et al. 2021 for an analysis of modes of resistance to these necropolitics in Brazil.

9    Cf. e.g. Molenaar and Praag 2022 for a discussion of the politics of the term vulnerability, with the term vulnerabilization emphasizing the need to think "vulnerability as the dynamic outcome of a process of 'vulnerabilisation' shaped by social order and power relations."

for example, orientalism,[10] xenophobia and racism, anti-Semitism, ageism, and ableism. According to Didier Fassin, "despite common perceptions, biopolitics does not proceed by one logic. It demonstrates a tension, inscribed in the body, between the supreme universality of life … and the exaltation of difference, for which biology offers an apparently insurmountable foundation … biopolitics is always a politics of otherness" (2001, 7). Such politics of otherness can take different and conflicting forms. This became, for instance, evident in the tensions that often characterized the treatment of elderly people during the pandemic, who were cast as one of the most vulnerable groups in need of protection, quarantined in care homes, and turned into mere statistics as hospital beds or deaths on the daily news. Their vulnerability sparked empathy and acts of genuine solidarity, at the same time that its mobilization in various political and media discourses ensured/comforted other parts of the population to be neither old nor vulnerable and endangered.

## Framing Bodies, Selves/Others, and Affects during COVID-19

Despite of or rather because of being a power that is "massifying, that is directed not as man-as-body but at man-as-species" (Foucault [1976] 1997, 243), biopower also affects the individual body. Foucault contrasts biopolitics, directed at the population and operating with models, statistics, and security mechanisms, to anatomo-politics or disciplinary power, directed at individual bodies, at "the body as a machine: its disciplining, the optimization of its capabilities, the extortion of its forces, the parallel increase of its usefulness and its docility, its integration into systems of efficient and economic controls at some points in his work" ([1978] 1990, 139). However, he emphasizes that these two forms of politics are in fact complementary, two poles of biopower, and it is due to "the play of technologies of discipline on the one hand and technologies of regulation on the other"—most evident in the element of the norm and the normalizing society—that biopower "succeeded in covering the whole surface that lies between the organic and the biological, between body and population" ([1976] 1997, 253).

The entanglements of individual bodies/anatomo-politics with the population or community/biopolitics, and moreover the entanglement of both forms

---

10    Only one infamous example is then US President Donald Trump labelling the virus the "Chinese virus."

of politics with the relations of self/Other also manifest in the evocation of discourses about immunity. As Roberto Esposito has shown in his influential work on immunity: "Whether the danger that lies in wait is a disease threatening the individual body, a violent intrusion into the body politic, or a deviant message entered the body electronic, what remains constant is the place where the threat is located, always on the border between the inside and the outside, between the self and the other, the individual and the common" (2011, 2). Similarly, Donna Haraway has argued that the immune system functions as "a map drawn to guide recognition and misrecognition of self and other in the dialects of Western biopolitics" (1991, 204). Originating as a legal and political term (Cohen 2009), "a political decision about privilege, in the sense of a law that applied only to certain classes of persons or individuals" (Neocleous 2022, 2), it was only in the nineteenth century that immunity entered the discourse of science and biomedicine, fused with that other political concept, self-defense. Since then, the notion of immunity-as-defense has influenced "how we imagine our bodies as living organisms but also how we imagine what it means to be an organism living among other organisms and what it means to be a human living among other humans" (Cohen 2009, 4). In an "age of immunology" (Napier 2003), the biopolitics of immunity-as-defense has persisted in form of an "immunity-security dispositif": During the coronavirus pandemic, "body and body politic were as one in their search for mutual security. We were encouraged to imagine the sovereign nation as a body and our body as a sovereign nation" (Neocleous 2022, 32). The military rhetoric employed by some politicians and journalists was only one manifestation of the notion of our bodies being under siege or in a 'war on COVID-19' (cf. also Ajana 2021). In this sense, little seems to have changed in the long history of the mobilization of military rhetoric in narratives of illness. As Susan Sontag has urged us, we should rethink metaphors of illness because the military metaphor, "overmobilizes, it overdescribes, and it powerfully contributes to the excommunicating and stigmatizing of the ill" (1990, 182).

The conflation of military and medical language is deeply ingrained in cultural discourses of immunity, though the notion of "immunity-as-defense" has been challenged from various sides (cf. Tauber 2000). As philosopher of immunology, Thomas Pradeu has argued, "such categories as 'defense,' 'repair,' and 'development' reflect more the way we, as investigators, address questions about bodily systems (and divide such processes into convenient categories) than real differences in nature" (2019, 10). Also feminist philosophers like Elizabeth Grosz with her notion of 'volatile bodies' (1994) or Margrit Shildrick with her concept of 'leaky bodies' (1997) have for a long time questioned the idea of a body with rigid boundaries, emphasizing instead its fluidity and permeability. The spread of the coronavirus pandemic repeatedly highlighted the ways in which human bodies are interconnected with other human bodies and also with non-human bodies, how they are part of larger ecological systems, as assemblages, i.e. "ever-changing human-nonhuman gatherings" (Lupton et al. 2021, 5; cf. De Landa 2006). And yet, essentialist and individualist notions of the self—connected to an ideal of a tightly controlled and regulated body—have often persisted to dominate the knowledge, practices and experiences of constitutions of self-hood, if not lived embodiment.[11] Discourses about COVID-19 have, once again, shown how the conflation of immunity and self-defense—against not-self—has often, though not without challenges and ambiguities, remained "the dominant, if often implicit, framework in which immunologists [and especially the larger public] conceive how the immune system works" (Pradeu 2019, 17). In the contemporary moment, the borders repeatedly (re)installed by the atomistic framework of the 'immune self' (cf. Tauber 1994)[12] and its metaphors of immunization (c.f. Esposito 2011; 2013) tend to resonate with nationalist and isolationist border politics as well as with contemporary neoliberal politics of responsibilization and capitalist interests in many places in the world.

All of these developments also point to the affective dimension of biopolitics. Biopower is so effective because it "works not only at the level of regulating reason and desire, but also in choreographing a repertoire of sensory stimulations" (Schuller 2018, 19). Emotions and feelings shape the ways in which individuals and communities experience and respond to crises like COVID-19. Moral panics accompanied the pandemic early on. In Germany, fears concerned decreasing productivity, decreasing mobility, decreasing consumption. Ironically, particularly in the early days of the pandemic, consumers themselves reacted with panic buying, hording toilet papers and hand sanitizers. Shuttered restaurants, theaters, cinemas, and opera houses, in turn, caused worries about the future of the cultural industry. Online classes and

---

11    Cf. also Ajana (2021) for a discussion of government's immunitary responses to the coronavirus pandemic.

12    Even the work of some critics and philosophers of biopolitics, according to Vanessa Lemm, is marked by a return of humanism – a belief in "the modern subject, a rational, social and moral agent capable of leading the revolution of the future" (2022, 150).

the concern for the education and the mental as well as physical health of children, at some points fostered crisis discourses about a 'lost generation.' Media reports about 'COVID 15,' i.e. the 15 extra pounds supposedly gained during quarantine, connected the COVID-19 pandemic with preexisting discourses about an 'obesity pandemic,' exacerbating weight stigma and furthering long-standing discourses of healthism and ableism. In the course of the pandemic, research showed that the COVID-19 pandemic has, indeed, had a profound impact on mental health and emotional well-being, as it lead to anxiety, stress, and depression.[13] These psychological responses have often been tied to the preventive biopolitical strategies such as quarantines, lockdowns, distance learning; they can also be linked to the widespread rhetoric of crisis and fear; and for some they may also have resulted from the medical condition of COVID-19 infections, the experience of living with post- and long-COVID or from the experiences of losing loved ones to the virus.

According to Sara Ahmed,

> In ... affective economies, emotions *do things*, and they align individuals with communities—or bodily space with social space—through the very intensity of their attachments. Rather than seeing emotions as psychological dispositions, we need to consider how they work, in concrete and particular ways, to mediate the relationship between the psychic and the social, between the individual and the collective." (2004, 119)

Emotions such as empathy, felt and mobilized at different points during the pandemic, have sparked shared moments of community, raising—sometimes short-lived—hopes for more substantial cultural changes (cf. Žižek 2020). These included intergenerational solidarity, outrage about haphazard health systems and global inequalities, systemic racism, climate change, gender inequalities and the realization that for many communities around the world quarantine, detention or surveillance are daily lived realities and not a state of exception. Then there were those experiencing the pandemic as a de-accelerator—allowing the privileged classes, in particular, more family time, more time at home, more 'quality time.' Global advertisement campaigns by Coke, Ikea, or McDonald's joined these discourses that sought to spread feelings

---

13    For meta-analysis of the effects of COVID-19 on mental health, cf. for example Cénat et al. 2022, Daniali, Martinussen, and Flaten 2023, Wu et al. 2021, Racine et al. 2021, and Leung et al. 2022.

of comfort and hope, evoking long-standing idealizations of family, home, community and, of course, consumption.

Among some social and political groups, fear and anxiety, in turn, seem to have exacerbated nationalist and racist tendencies, already on the rise before the pandemic, and contributed to the widening of social divides. The complexities of pandemic biopolitics, othering, and affect become particularly evident if we take into account how various protest movements have fused criticisms of government regulations, anti-vaccination policies, conspiracy narratives, and right-wing agendas. In Germany, the violence of some of these alignments became visible when a week before the symposium that initiated this volume, a coronavirus sceptic shot a young gas station clerk when the latter asked him to wear his mask. Movements and ideologies such as the US rooted QAnon or the German *Querdenker* frame themselves as critical responses to governmental biopolitics, which they cast as a totalitarian grasp onto life. As they seek to resist this grasp, they put forward alternative narratives about the pandemic, fused with conspiracy narratives and rhetoric of othering. According to Michael Butter and Peter Knight,

> [W]hile there is a great variety in the specific strains of conspiracy narratives that emerged and mutated since the initial outbreak, they often express a core belief that 'they' (the government, the health authorities, the mainstream media, the global elite, the leaders of powerful nations like China or the United States, etc.) are lying to 'us' (the ordinary people, the members of a specific nation, ethnicity, culture, or religion, etc.). (2023)

In their articulation of resistance against this perceived illegitimate control, many of these narratives function as post-truth politics that align with long-standing discriminatory discourses. These historically and geographically specific, yet increasingly globally widespread patterns show that definitions of the Other may be contingent and can be instrumentalized by various groups and discursive formations to different effects.

## The Ambiguity of Biopolitics in a Pandemic World

Biopolitics is neither one coherent technology of power, nor does biopower operate as if a centralized power aimed for the production of a specific form of subjecthood. Biopolitics rather produces as its effects notions of subjectivity, as it modulates discourses, practices, forms and experiences of embodiment with different and often ambiguous outcomes. In the words of Michael Dillon and Luis Lobo-Guerro: "[I]t is a complex array of changing mechanisms concerned with regulating the contingent economy of species life. Identity may follow from this, but identity production is not its initial driver" (2008, 268). Biopower operates as mechanisms of security regulating processes of circulation "in the very broad sense of movement, exchange, and contact, as form of dispersion, and also as form of distribution" (Foucault [1978] 2007, 64). In contrast to the juridical mechanism and the disciplinary mechanism, the apparatus of security does not primarily prohibit or prescribe, though it may use "some instruments of prescription and prohibition" ([1978] 2007, 47); "the essential function of security ... is to respond to a reality in such a way that this response cancels out the reality to which it responds—nullifies it, or limits, checks, or regulates it. ... [T]his regulation within the element of reality is fundamental in apparatuses of security" ([1978] 2007, 47). For Foucault this also means that the liberal notion of "freedom is nothing else but the correlative of the deployment of apparatuses of security" ([1978] 2007, 48). Taking these notions of modulation—which are central to Foucault's understanding of biopower— seriously, allows a nuanced perspective on biopolitical technologies of governmentality. This includes the understanding of their overlap with technologies of disciplinary power such as surveillance, restrictions and other mechanisms aimed at the production of docile bodies, but also the acknowledgment that—as Foucault put it in an interview—"not everything is bad, but ... everything is dangerous, which is not exactly the same as bad. If everything is dangerous, then we always have something to do" ([1983] 2003, 104).[14]

Biopolitical measures implemented during the COVID-19 pandemic to limit the spread of the virus evoke various meanings, functions, effects, and affects. By supplementing Foucauldian approaches to governmentality and biopolitics with assemblage theory and more-than-human theory, scholars such as Deborah Lupton et al. (2021) and Gay Hawkins (2022), have started to show this for instance with regards to mass masking (Lupton et al. 2021) and social distancing (Hawkins 2022). Masks, as Lupton and colleagues conclude,

---

14    The quote is part of a conversation between Foucault, Paul Rabinow and Hubert Dreyfus from 1983.

[P]rotect us from nonhuman entities such as the novel coronavirus, but simultaneously have sociomaterial effects on the environment and ecosystem. They are things that come together with human bodies, other living and non-living things, place and space to generate forms of safety, self-expression, embodied socialities, creativity and care but also disturbing affective forces such as anger, frustration, discomfort, racism, social exclusion and shame. (2021, 85)

Hawkins frames social distancing as being "not about contestation or war with the virus—erecting borders and effective separation—but rather inherent co-operation with it" (2022, 125). Social distancing, he suggests, "is not a behavioural response to risk, to a new and threatening environment; it is a practical action that makes a contagious situation real and establishes forms of local order within it. It is evidence of how suggestion and co-operation become implicated in the administration of life" (2022, 126).

Seeking to challenge a specific canon of criticism of biopolitics, there have also been attempts to formulate an affirmative stance towards biopolitics; for example by Benjamin Bratton who, in a direct response to Giorgio Agamben's negative stance towards biopolitics and COVID-19 regulations, articulates the need for a "positive biopolitics"; a "post-pandemic politics" that is "inclusive, materialist, restorative, rationalist, based on a demystified image of the human species, anticipating a future different from the one prescribed by many cultural traditions" (2022). Sergei Prozorov has called for a democratization of biopolitical governance, with democracy understood as "the way to affirm life in the myriad ways of living" (2019, 200). And according to Karsten Schubert, "democratic biopolitics understood normatively, consists of the critical analysis of differentiated vulnerabilities with the aim of easing the inequalities through political measures. The key would be to avoid regulations that reinforce existing structures of discrimination, as often happened during the coronavirus pandemic" (2022, 102).

A closer discussion of these positions clearly goes beyond the scope of this introduction, but the book is positioned in these debates in so far as it seeks to use the concepts of biopolitics and othering to scrutinize the ambivalent mechanisms, modulations, and effects of biopower. In this it is in line with Chris Hall's reasoning:

We must think biopolitically, ambivalently, about the global populations affected by accumulating vaccine stockpiles, about lives rendered disposable through anti-masking and anti-vaccination rhetorics of freedom, about science's retrenchment as supposed fount of objective truth. We can do any of this productively only by starting from the knowledge that such forces, and the politics they shape, preserve more than survival as they both save and oppress, and not along lines that are set or clearly discernable. (2022)

Taken together, the following chapters—which originate from different academic disciplines, focus on a variety of historical, geographical, cultural and medical contexts, and offer different, maybe at times even conflicting, arguments—may hopefully add a small and humble piece to the big mosaic of historical and cultural studies of pandemics, biopolitics and othering already published or still needed. Epidemics cannot be framed as linear narratives (cf. Charters and Heitman 2021), as perhaps some movies and a lot of public and political rhetoric suggests. Although a vaccine was discovered for COVID-19 and masks and social distancing as visible signifiers of the pandemic have increasingly been removed in many countries, COVID-19 has already begun to show that an epidemic tends to develop into a cyclical event or endemic disease (Charters and Heitman 2021) that might have come to an end for one social group but not for others. By focusing not only on the contemporary moment, or rather by putting it into relation, conversation, and contrast to historical events and developments of pandemics/epidemics in their various and specific historical and glocal contexts, the following essays aim at creating, facilitating and further nuancing interdisciplinary academic discussions about the manifold manifestations and impacts of biopolitics and othering in epidemics and their discursive formations.

## Historical and Cultural Perspectives on Epidemics and the (Bio)Politics of Othering

The contributions to this volume offer a number of historical and cultural perspectives on the relations of pandemics/epidemics, biopolitics and othering by authors with backgrounds in history, political science, theology, Romance studies, American studies, East Asian studies, anthropology, clinical education, cultural studies, postcolonial studies, queer studies, literary studies, and media studies. Many of these contributions explore histories of epidemics with a particular focus on the interrelations of biopolitics and othering in the context of (post)colonialism, while others pay particular attention to the ways in which processes of othering in times of pandemics are closely linked to specific media and forms of representation. All of them elucidate how biopolitics and othering manifest in specific cultural historical contexts, (re)produce specific structures of knowledge and power, and affect individual and communal bodies along the intersection of various axes of social differentiation.

Romana Radlwimmer's contribution compares colonial texts from the time of the Spanish colonization of Mexico and contemporary COVID-19 fiction from the Romance-speaking world to explore the historical and textual continuites in the ways these very different texts frame the position of the (post)colonial Other. According to Radlwimmer, a comparison reveals the long-lasting impact of colonial knowledge-power that manifests itself in stories that accompany the (post)colonial biopolitics of illness in discrepant ways, depending on the position of the speaker. Martin Gabriel zooms in on the colonial management of and the biopolitical measures taken against the historical outbreaks of smallpox in Guatemala and Oxaca (Mexico) towards the end of the eighteenth century. As Gabriel's historical study reveals, while in both cases these measures primarily targeted Indigenous populations, the strategies and the outcomes differed; as did the framing of the non-European as cultural Other. Anke Scherer's contribution shifts the focus to South East Asia and explores proceses of othering in the context of Japan's colonization of Taiwan. Specifically, her study focuses on the campaigns of the Japanese colonial government to stop the plague in the 1910s, to elucidate how the newly developed concept of hygienic modernity as opposed to traditional Chinese medicine functioned as a device of othering in the framing of the Taiwanese population.

Claudia Jahnel's contribution zooms out again and offers broader reflections on the strategies of othering in the context of (post)colonial development studies in general and global health discourses in the context of COVID-19 in particular. By exploring the demarcation of borders and boundaries and the politics of emotion, Jahnel shows how COVID-19 has reinforced global hierarchies and inequalities, thereby securing the domination of the Global North, while her analyses also shed light on possibilities to shatter Eurocentric models of charity and future-making. Danielle Heberle Viegas examines the continuing influences of colonial imaginaries and racial hierarchies on patterns of spatial mobility in Brazil during the COVID-19 pandemic. Specifically, Viegas shows how the increase in nature tourism and the demand for subdivisions in gated communities are rooted in particular biopolitical histories and linked to (utopian) notions of Brazilian tropicality. The next chapter explores the complex dynamics of othering in the history of epidmics/pandemics, by turning from governmental biopolitics to conspiracy narratives. Martin Tschiggerl's contribution traces the historical roots of othering in COVID-19 conspiracy theories in the German-speaking world. By comparing anti-vaccination conspiracy theories that emerged in the wake of smallpox in the late nineteenth/early twentieth century with those that were spread during the COVID-19 pandemic, his contribution reveals the ideological continuity between radical opposition to vaccination and anti-Semitic conspiracy theories.

Martin Lüthe's contribution takes its cue from discourses about a pandemic beneath the pandemic, namely cultural anxieties about 'covbesity', i.e. an 'obesity' pandemic related to the COVID-19 pandemic. Drawing on disability studies and fat studies, Lüthe explores discourses about fatness in a U.S. American and German context, and focuses on their links to discourses about digital gaming. As his contribution shows, anxieties regarding body shape and physical fitness are frequently negotiated through the on-screen bodies and the off-screen bodies of digital games and digital sport games. By looking specifically at the relation of pandemics and media in the context of a (re)presentational shift brought about by COVID-19, Julia Eckel and Elisa Linseisen discuss questions of presence. These questions, they argue, have become virulent due to the spatial/physical presence of people as a main risk of contagion on the one hand and the increased need for forms of mediated presence on the other hand. In their contribution, they explore the changed qualities of presence that have developed in the context of videoconferencing tools in their relatedness to both digital media and structural intertwinements with forms of (digital) othering. Natalie Pielok explores the concept and practice of breathing as an essential bodily practice that is not available to all people in the same way and that opens up questions about structural politics that allow lives, bodies and places to breathe differently. During the COVID-19 pandemic the practice of breathing has become especially visible when breathing was disrupted. In her contribution, Pielok analyzes 'the scream' as mobilized in audio-visual installations and performances to explore the resistant and affective potential of breathing from the perspective of media and sound studies, queer theory, and Black studies.

The book closes in dialogical form, as four scholars from different disciplinary and cultural backgrounds share their perspectives on the (in)comparability of HIV/AIDS and SARS-CoV-2/COVID-19. By debating and highlighting the significance of the AIDS pandemic in light of its differences to the

COVID-19 pandemic, Simon Dickel, Roselyne Masamha, Lennon Mhishi and Florian Zitzelsberger, emphasize the need for differentiating views, and draw particular attention to the significance of AIDS in relation to processes of sexual and racial stigmatization. At the same time, their exchange highlights important aspects, also to be taken into account and explored when critically analyzing pandemic biopolitics and processes of othering in the context of COVID-19. The exchange presents both a thought-provoking closure to this volume and an important starting point for further research.

## Works Cited

Ahmed, Sara. 2004. "Affective Economies." *Social Text* 22, no. 2 (Summer): 117–39.

Ajana, Bithaj. 2021. "Immunitarianism: Defence and Sacrifice in the Politics of Covid-19." *History and Philosophy of the Life Sciences* 43, no. 25 (February). https://doi.org/10.1007/s40656-021-00384-9.

Bhabha, Homi K. 1983. "The Other Question…" *Screen* 24, no. 6: 18–36.

Bratton, Benjamin. (2021) 2022. *The Revenge of the Real: Politics for a Post-Pandemic World*. London: Verso. Kindle.

Butler, Judith. 1993. *Bodies That Matter: On the Discursive Limits of Sex*. London: Routledge.

———. 2020. "Capitalism Has Its Limits: Judith Butler Discuss [*sic*] the COVID-19 Pandemic, and Its Escalating Political and Social Effects in America." *Verso Books* (blog). March 30, 2020. https://www.versobooks.com/blogs/4603-capitalism-has-its-limits.

Butter, Michael, and Peter Knight. 2023. "Introduction: COVID-19 Conspiracy Narratives in Global Perspective." In *Covid Conspiracy Narratives in Global Perspective*, edited by Michael Butter and Peter Knight. New York: Routledge. Kindle.

Cavalcanti Muniz, Renata, Fiorella Macchiavello Ferradas, Georgina M. Gomez, and Lee J. Pegler. 2021. "Covid-19 in Brazil in an Era of Necropolitics: Resistance in the Face of Disaster." *Disasters* 45, no. S1: S97–S118.

Cénat, Jude Mary, Seyed Mohammad Mahdi Moshirian Farahi, Rose Darly Dalexis, Wina Paul Darius, Farid Mansoub Bekarkhanechi, Hannah Poisson, Cathy Broussard, Gloria Ukwu, Emmanuelle Auguste, Duy Dat Nguyen, Ghizlène Sehabi, Sarah Elizabeth Furyk, Andi Phaelle Gedeon, Olivia Onesi, Aya Mesbahi El Aouame, Samiyah Noor Khodabocus,

Muhammad S. Shah, and Patrick R. Labelle. 2022. "The Global Evolution of Mental Health Problems during the COVID-19 Pandemic: A Systematic Review and Meta-Analysis of Longitudinal Studies." *Journal of Affective Disorders* 315 (October): 70–95.

Charters, Erica, and Kristin Heitman. 2021. "How Epidemics End." *Centaurus* 63, no. 1: 210–24.

Christiaens, Tim. 2021. "Biomedical Technocracy, the Networked Public Sphere and the Biopolitics of COVID-19: Notes on the Agamben Affair." *Culture, Theory, and Critique* 62, no. 4: 404–21.

Christiaens, Tim, and Stijn De Cauwer. 2020. "The Biopolitics of Immunity in Times of COVID-19: An Interview with Roberto Esposito." *Antipode Online.* June 16, 2020. https://antipodeonline.org/2020/06/16/interview-with-rob erto-esposito/.

Cohen, Ed. 2009. *A Body Worth Defending: Immunity, Biopolitics, and the Apotheosis of the Modern Body.* Durham: Duke University Press.

Daniali, Hojjat, Monica Martinussen, and Magne Arve Flaten. 2023. "A Global Meta-Analysis of Depression, Anxiety, and Stress Before and during COVID-19." *Health Psychology* 42, no. 2: 124–38. https://doi.org/10.1037/he a0001259.

de Beauvoir, Simone. (1948) 2010. *The Second Sex.* London: Vintage Books.

De Landa, Manuel. 2006. *A New Philosophy of Society: Assemblage Theory and Social Complexity.* London: Continuum.

Dillon, Michael, and Luis Lobo-Guerrero. 2008. "Biopolitics of Security in the 21st Century: An Introduction." *Review of International Studies* 34, no. 2: 265–92.

Downs, Jim. 2021. *Maladies of Empire: How Colonialism, Slavery, and War Transformed Medicine.* Cambridge: Harvard University Press.

Eichelberger, Laura. 2007. "SARS and New York's Chinatown: The Politics of Risk and Blame during an Epidemic of Fear." *Social Science & Medicine* 65, no. 6: 1284–95.

Esposito, Roberto. 2011. *Immunitas: The Protection and Negation of Life.* Cambridge: Polity Press.

———. 2013. *Terms of the Political: Community, Immunity, Biopolitics.* New York: Fordham University Press.

Fassin, Didier. 2001. "The Biopolitics of Otherness: Undocumented Foreigners and Racial Discrimination in French Public Debate." *Anthropology Today* 17, no. 1 (February): 3–7.

Foucault, Michel. (1976) 1997. *'Society Must Be Defended': Lectures at the Collège de France, 1975–1976*. Edited by Mauro Bertani and Alesandro Fontana. New York: Picador.

———. (1978) 2007. *Security, Territory, Population: Lectures at the Collège de France, 1977–1978*. Edited by Michel Senellart. New York: Palgrave Macmillan.

———. (1978) 1990. *The History of Sexuality: An Introduction*. New York: Vintage Books.

———. (1983) 2003. "On the Genealogy of Ethics: An Overview of Work in Progress." In *The Essential Foucault: Selections from The Essential Works of Foucault 1954–1984*, edited by Paul Rabinow and Nikolas Rose, 102–25. New York: The New Press.

Grosz, Elizabeth. 1994. *Volatile Bodies: Toward a Corporeal Feminism*. Bloomington: Indiana University Press.

Hall, Chris. 2022. "Ambivalent Thinking amid Pandemic Biopolitics." *European Journal of Political Theory*. https://doi.org/10.1177/14748851221143450.

Haraway, Donna. 1988. "Situated Knowledges: The Science Question in Feminism and the Privilege of Partial Perspective." *Feminist Studies* 14, no. 3: 575–99.

———. 1991. *Simians, Cyborgs, and Women: The Reinvention of Nature*. New York: Routledge.

Hardt, Michael, and Antonio Negri. 2001. *Empire*. Cambridge: Harvard University Press.

Hawkins, Gay. 2022. "The Micropolitics of Social Distancing: Habit, Contagion and the Suggestive Realm." In *The Viral Politics of Covid-19: Nature, Home, and Planetary Health*, edited by Vanessa Lemm and Miguel Vatter, 113–28. Singapore: Palgrave Macmillan.

Hill Collins, Patricia. 1990. *Black Feminist Thought: Knowledge, Consciousness, and the Politics of Empowerment*. Boston: Unwin Hyman.

hooks, bell. 1984. *Feminist Theory from Margin to Center*. Boston: South End Press.

Howard, Mark. 2022. "The Necropolice Economy: Mapping Biopolitical Priorities and Human Expendability in the Time of COVID-19." *Societies* 12, no. 2. https://doi.org/10.3390/soc12010002.

Jáuregui, Carlos A., and David Solodkow. 2018. "Biopolitics and the Farming (of) Life in Bartolomé de las Casas." *Studies in the History of Christian Traditions* 189: 127–66.

Kupfer, Antonia, and Constanze Stutz, eds. 2022. *Covid, Crisis, Care, and Change? International Gender Perspectives on Re/Production, State and Feminist Transitions*. Opladen: Verlag Barbara Budrich.

Laterza, Vito, and Louis Philippe Romer. 2020. "Coronavirus, Herd Immunity and the Eugenics of the Market." *Aljazeera: Opinions.* April 14, 2020. https://www.aljazeera.com/indepth/opinion/coronavirus-herd-immunity-eugenics-market-200414104531234.html.

Lemm, Vanessa. 2022. "Ideologies of Contagion and Communities of Life." In *The Viral Politics of Covid-19: Nature, Home, and Planetary Health,* edited by Vanessa Lemm and Miguel Vatter, 145–60. Singapore: Palgrave Macmillan.

Leung, Candi M. C., Margaret K. Ho, Alina A. Bharwani, Hugo Cogo-Moreira, Yishan Wang, Mathew S. C. Chow, Xiaoyan Fan, Sandro Galea, Gabriel M. Leung, and Michael Y. Ni. 2022. "Mental Disorders Following COVID-19 and Other Epidemics: A Systematic Review and Meta-Analysis." *Translational Psychiatry* 12 (May): 205.

Li, Yao, and Harvey L. Nicholson Jr. 2021. "When 'Model Minorities' Become 'Yellow Peril'—Othering and the Racialization of Asian Americans in the COVID-19 Pandemic." *Sociology Compass* 15, no. 2: e12849. https://doi.org/10.1111/soc4.12849.

Lorenzini, Daniele. 2021. "Biopolitics in the Time of Coronavirus." *Critiqual Inquiry* 47, no. S2: S40–S45.

Lupton, Deborah, Clare Southerton, Marianne Clark, and Ash Watson. 2021. *The Face Mask in COVID Times: A Sociomaterial Analysis.* Berlin: De Gruyter.

Mbembe, Achille. 2003. "Necropolitics." *Public Culture* 15, no. 1: 11–40.

———. 2019. *Necropolitics.* Durham: Duke University Press.

Meloni, Maurizio. 2022. "A Foucauldian Moment or the Longue Durée? COVID-19 in Context." In *The Viral Politics of Covid-19: Nature, Home, and Planetary Health,* edited by Vanessa Lemm and Miguel Vatter, 53–72. Singapore: Palgrave Macmillan.

Molenaar, Jil, and Lore Van Praag. 2022. "Migrants as 'Vulnerable Groups' in the COVID-19 Pandemic: A Critical Discourse Analysis of a Taken-for-Granted Label in Academic Literature." *SSM—Qualitative Research in Health* 2 (December). https://doi.org/10.1016/j.ssmqr.2022.100076.

Napier, David A. 2003. *The Age of Immunology: Conceiving a Future in an Alienating World.* Chicago: The University of Chicago Press.

Navarro, Sharon A., and Samantha L. Hernandez. 2022. *The Color of Covid-19: The Racial Inequality of Marginalized Communities.* New York: Routledge.

Neocleous, Mark. 2022. *The Politics of Immunity: Security and the Policing of Bodies.* London: Verso Book.

Pradeu, Thomas. 2019. *Philosophy of Immunology.* Cambridge: Cambridge University Press.

Prozorov, Sergei. 2019. *Democratic Biopolitics: Popular Sovereignty and the Power of Life*. Edinburgh: Edinburgh University Press.

Quinan, C. L., and Kathrin Thiele, eds. 2020. "Biopolitics, Necropolitics, Cosmopolitics—Feminist and Queer Interventions: An Introduction." *Journal of Gender Studies* 29, no. 1: 1–8.

Racine, Nicole, Rachel Eirich, Jessica Cooke, Jenney Zhu, Paolo Pador, Nicole Dunewold, and Sheri Madigan. 2021. "When the Bough Breaks: A Systematic Review and Meta-Analysis of Mental Health Symptoms in Mothers of Young Children during the COVID-19 Pandemic." *Infant Mental Health Journal* 43 (September): 36–54. https://doi.org/10.1002/imhj.21959.

Said, Edward. 1978. *Orientalism*. New York: Vintage Books.

Sarasin, Philipp. 2020. "Understanding the Coronavirus Pandemic with Foucault?" *Genealogy+Critique* (blog). March 31, 2020. https://blog.genealogy-critique.net/essays/254/understanding-corona-with-foucault.

Schubert, Karsten. 2020. "Crying for Repression: Populist and Democratic Biopolitics in Times of COVID-19." *Critical Legal Thinking*. April 1, 2020. https://criticallegalthinking.com/2020/04/01/crying-for-repression-populist-and-democratic-biopolitics-in-times-of-covid-19/.

———. 2022. "Biopolitics of COVID-19: Capitalist Continuities and Democratic Openings." *Interalia—A Journal for Queer Studies* 16: 95–105.

Schuller, Kyla. 2018. *The Biopolitics of Feeling: Race, Sex, and Science in the Nineteenth Century*. Durham: Duke University Press.

Shildrick, Margrit. 1997. *Leaky Bodies and Boundaries: Feminism, Postmodernism and (Bio)ethics*. London: Routledge.

Sontag, Susan. 1990. *Illness as Metaphor and AIDS and Its Metaphors*. New York: Anchor.

Sparke, Matthew, and Dimitar Anguelov. 2020. "Contextualizing Coronavirus Geographically." *Transactions of the Institute of British Geographers* 45, no. 3: 498–508.

Spivak, Gayatri Chakravorty. 1985. "The Rani of Sirmur: An Essay in Reading the Archives." *History and Theory* 24, no. 3: 247–72.

Tauber, Alfred I. 1994. *The Immune Self: Theory or Metaphor?* Cambridge: Cambridge University Press.

———. 2000. "Moving Beyond the Immune Self?" *Seminars in Immunology* 12, no. 3 (June): 241–8.

UN WOMEN. 2020. "From Insight to Action: Gender Equality in the Wake of Covid-19." https://www.unwomen.org/sites/default/files/Headquarters/A

ttachments/Sections/Library/Publications/2020/Gender-equality-in-the-wake-of-COVID-19-en.pdf.

World Health Organization. 2020a. "COVID-19 Public Health Emergency of International Concern (PHEIC) Global Research and Innovation Forum." February 12, 2020. https://www.who.int/publications/m/item/covid-19-public-health-emergency-of-international-concern-(pheic)-global-research-and-innovation-forum.

———. 2020b. "WHO Director-General's Opening Remarks at the Media Briefing on COVID-19—11 March 2020." March 11, 2020. https://www.who.int/director-general/speeches/detail/who-director-general-s-opening-remarks-at-the-media-briefing-on-covid-19---11-march-2020.

———. 2023. "WHO Coronavirus (COVID-19) Dashboard." Last accessed April 3, 2023. https://covid19.who.int/.

Wu, Tianchen, Xiaoqian Jia, Huifeng Shi, Jieqiong Niu, Xiaohan Yin, Jialei Xie, and Xiaoli Wang. 2021. "Prevalence of Mental Health Problems during the COVID-19 Pandemic: A Systematic Review and Meta-Analysis." *Journal of Affective Disorders* 281 (February): 91–8.

Žižek, Slavoj. 2020. "Der Mensch wird nicht mehr derselbe gewesen sein: Das ist die Lektion, die das Coronavirus für uns bereithält." *NZZ*. March 13, 2020. https://www.nzz.ch/feuilleton/coronavirus-der-mensch-wird-nie-mehr-derselbe-gewesen-sein-ld.154625.

## 2. Pandemics, Biopolitics and Coloniality: From Chronicles of the Indies to COVID-19 Fictions

*Romana Radlwimmer*

In his 2020 photo series *The Luxury of Social Isolation*, Gui Christ documents the COVID-19 crisis in one of the largest São Paulo favelas, Paraisópolis, where 150,000 people live crammed together, forced to share water supplies and to go to work. Antithetically, the favela's inhabitants appear isolated, in empty, chaotic surroundings, such as the woman in an arbitrarily built house (fig. 1).[1]

Like other subjects of Christ's photographs, she is positioned in the central vertical axis of the image; the ladder she stands on prolongs her figure. The horizontal vanishing lines of the patio to the right and to the left of the ladder vaguely sketch the silhouette of a cross, which is repeated in the rose and the letters printed on the woman's black shirt, connecting to Christian pictography, and situating her, like the other depicted persons, symbolically in the place of Jesus' passion. The portrayed are Brazilians of African descent, who, according to statistics, represented a vulnerable ethnic group highly affected by COVID-19 (Ferreira and Camargo 2021, 1). Their masks cover their mouths and thus, hinder their ability to speak (Spivak 1994, 83), but their eyes are firmly focused on the camera. Gui Christ's series wins the third prize in the Harvard David-Rockefeller-Center's Competition *Documenting the Impact of Covid-19 through Photography: Collective Isolation in Latin America*. From a center of global knowledge production, Christ presents and exploits the gaze onto

1   This research is sponsored by the Volkswagen Foundation in the framework of my project "Pandemics and Coloniality: Biopolitical Entanglements in Early Modern Chronicles and COVID-19 Narratives" http://portal.volkswagenstiftung.de/search/proj ectDetails.do?ref=98771. I would like to thank my scientific team for the data collected for this article (in alphabetical order): Cosima Ballmann, Tim Balke, Katja Keßler, and Moritz Mainka.

the Other. He, and the spectator, are not part of the favela, but look at the inhabitants' stereotypical misery. And yet, his images interrupt the view from a "rational" North onto an "irrational" South (Adorno 1988, 64), as they self-consciously perform this gaze onto the Other. The frontal perspective on all subjects inhibits mimetic illusion: the observers are not part of a conversation, but have to stare, alienated, at the subjects' silence and at their own look at the Other, while the Other looks back at them through dark-skinned, covered faces or through the eye-like windows of shanty town's red-brick buildings and dirty white high-rises, containing that in Paraisópolis, social isolation is a luxury. As Christ's images stage the marginal space, the own physical persona is the commodity to circulate in society in the face of "bare" survival (Agamben 1998, 42, 97); the social restrictions advised by the WHO cannot grant the right to live.

*Figure 1: Gui Christ:* The Luxury of Social Isolation *(2020).*

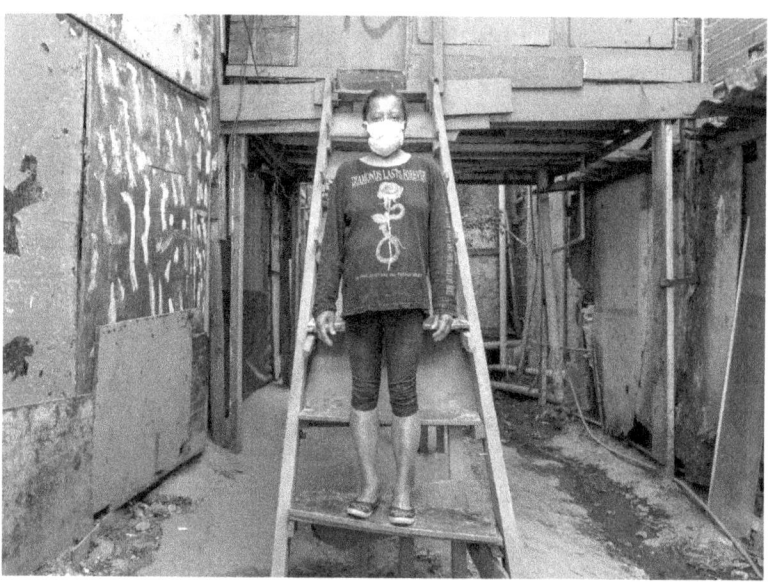

Even before COVID-19, death in Paraisópolis was quantified in numbers, and hardly ever appeared as a narrative of individual mourning; news about, for instance, "9 deceased" in a police intervention were habitual, and the sanitary crisis reinforced this representation (Safatle 2020). Even if all quarantines are, according to Boaventura de Sousa Santos, discriminatory, they are even more so to the "South of the quarantine," in the spatio-temporally defined politics of suffering where the cultural and social Other is constructed (De Sousa Santos 2020, 45). Figurations like the favela paradigmatically connect to an (often racist and classist) othering, and the 2020 pandemic nudged a research trend to read such practices in terms of coloniality (the long shadows of colonialism) and biopolitics (the power over life) or—as in the case of Brazil—necropolitics (the production of death). This tendency to connect the pandemic with coloniality and biopolitics (Safatle 2020, Alencar Jr. 2020, Caponi 2021, Pereira Campos dos Santos et al. 2020, Silva 2020, Tommaselli 2020) centrally asks how COVID-19 has created a "painful scenario in which some human creatures assert their rights to live at the expense of others, re-inscribing the spurious distinction between grievable and ungrievable lives" (Butler 2020). According to concepts of coloniality, sixteenth-century expansionism generated—and excluded—the colonial Other which structurally still exists in contemporary societies and thinking (Quijano 2014, 777–9). In postcolonial contexts, phenomena of othering during COVID-19 have been associated with the colonial past, connecting them to early modern manifestations of disease. Activists who feared a native "genocide" (Bragato et al. 2020; Chervenski Figueira et al. 2020) in today's Latin America replayed the discourse of the extinction of entire populations through imported epidemics which supposedly enabled sixteenth-century military success (Vainfas 2020, Brooks 2003).

Both scenarios, the contemporary and the historic, can be read as biopolitical interventions which define the space given to the human body and spirit (Foucault 1976, 179–83). Michel Foucault, who coined the term "biopolitics," investigated how racism developed in colonial setting as the basis for future biopolitics to justify the killing of people ([1997] 2003, 257). Achille Mbembe believes that necropolitics—the production of death—practices forms of othering that connect early to late modern coloniality: "The perception of the existence of the Other as ... danger whose biophysical elimination would strengthen my potential to life ... is one of the many imaginaries of sovereignty characteristic of both early and late modernity itself" (Mbembe 2003, 18). Mbembe sees processes of othering inherited from the colonial period as ongoing biopolitical patterns which are "translating the social conflicts of the industrial world in racial terms" and thus "ended up comparing the working classes and 'stateless people' of the industrial world to the 'savages' of the colonial world" (2003, 18). While Mbembe stresses that colonial structures shape today's necropolitics, Carlos Jáuregui and David Solodkov apply biopolitical thought to sixteenth-century colonialism and affirm that "colonial designs for governing life and exploiting work were not 'precursors' to biopolitics; they were fully biopolitical. ...Through plans to manage and govern the indigenous and African populations and to exploit their bodies, colonialism in America constituted a vast laboratory of modern biopolitics" (2019, 132). The proposed reciprocity between the former colonies and postcolonial societies is at the center of this article which investigates the language and practices that accompany the biopolitics of illness. The analyzed texts are Chronicles of the Indies—Bernal Díaz del Castillo's *Historia verdadera*, the Florentine Codex, and a reprinted sermon by António Vieira—and their intersections with COVID-19 fiction—Daniel Galera's short novels compiled in *O deus das avancas* (2021) and Valter Hugo Mãe's novel *As doenças do Brasil* (2021). Together, these texts prove the long-lasting effects of colonial knowledge-power which manifests across historical times, geographical space, traveling through different media and genres.

## The Contagious Other

In 2021, as all eyes were set on the Corona pandemic, Mexico's government also commemorated the 500 years of the fall of Tenochitlán, the Aztec capital which the Spanish conquered after only two years of siege ("Los ecos" 2021). The Spanish military success was preceded by the smallpox epidemics in the Mexica nation in 1520 (Crosby [1986] 2015, 200), exactly half a millennium before the outbreak of the Corona virus. Spanish chronicles narrate how even after 1521, the illness caused local rulers to surrender to Hernán Cortés: "[E]n aquel tiempo anduvo la viruela tan común en la Nueva España, fallescían muchos caciques, y sobre a quién pertenescía el cacicazgo ..., venían a Cortes, como a señor asoluto de toda la tierra, para que por su mano e autoridad alzase por señor a quien le pertenescía" [sic] (In those days, smallpox commonly went about in New Spain, and many caciques died, and those who inherited the leadership came to Cortés, the absolute ruler of the entire territory, for his hand and authority were to assign as ruler those who owned this title) (Díaz del Castillo 2015, 519).[2] After conquest, the imported illnesses form part of the newly es-

2    In this article, all translations from Spanish or Portuguese which are not referenced are mine.

tablished colonial societies and cement the imperial hierarchy which arises out of the "discovery *self* makes of the *other*" in the so-called "discovery of America" (Todorov [1982] 1999, 3; italics in original). Spanish chroniclers construct the contagious Other not only in the high native death toll and its consequences of military surrender, they also blame an African slave to have brought the virus to America in the first place (Díaz del Castillo 2015, 456). The narrative of the contagious Other is persistent and soon becomes part of popular culture, as in seventeenth-century interior decorations. *Biombos* or household folding screens, for instance, pictographically retell the story of the first porter of the plague, who is easily recognizable through his dark skin color and who is being punished on the images (Martínez del Río de Redo 2005, 130).

In the sixteenth century, Mexico's pre-Columbian writing and painting traditions blend with Spanish impulses into culturally 'hybrid' formats. These native accounts take a stance on what imperial illness means to them, contesting the newly established biopolitical order that administered and controlled the colonized Other. Many of these codices were produced by Mexica for Mexica and about the Mexica (Townsend 2017, 1). The Florentine Codex, "the single most well-developed and well-known" (Lockhart 1993, 5) Nahua account, was compiled by Bernardino de Sahagún and his *tlacuilos*, a team of Nahua writers and artists. Two generations after conquest, Nahua interviewers and interpreters recorded the collective memory of their elders who had experienced conquest. Written in Nahuatl and in Spanish, and illustrated by almost 2000 images, the codex partly interferes with and partly continues the tradition of Nahua pictographic annals.[3] The Codex exemplifies the ideological battles between the Crown's and the church's biopolitical forces and their subversion. Sahagún's text repeats the rhetoric of the church; however, the Spanish words stand equally next to Nahuatl, and the two languages not always express the same perspective on phenomena. They are complemented by native illustrations which tell an alternative story from the Mexica point of view (Favrot Peterson 2019, 30). Sahagún's project is at times supported by the Crown; however, the imperial rules shift and in 1577, "Felipe II. ordered the confiscation of all writings related to the Indies and Indians" (Rao 2019, 38). Hence, the book is never published and, moreover, is in danger of disappearing completely (Adorno 1988, 62; Spagnesi 1993; Terraciano 2019, 2).

---

3    For a comprehensive general introduction to the Códice Florentino see Terraciano (2019).

The Codex is written between the two infectious plagues of 1545 and 1576, and in his prologues, Sahagún reflects on the illnesses' devastating consequences for the indigenous population which he had witnessed with his own eyes (Malvido and Viesca 1985, 27). Chapter 29 of Florentine Codex's Book 12—the book on the conquest—remembers how the Spanish imported the virus. It shows how the first smallpox plague measured life in the city during the siege of 1520 and how it prepared Spanish victory. In this panorama, the notion of the Other is caught in the tensions constructed by the Nahuatl and the Spanish text, which differ from one another. James Lockhart's brilliant critical edition of Florentine Codex' Book 12 translates both the Nahuatl and the Spanish text into English, and thus, facilitates a cross-reading of the representations of the "contagious Other" in both languages. The Nahuatl text reads as follows:

> Twenty-ninth chapter, where it is said how, at the time the Spaniards left Mexico, there came an illness of pustules of which many local people died; it was called 'the great rash' [smallpox]. Before the Spaniards appeared to us, first an epidemic broke out, a sickness of pustules. It began in Tepeihuitl. Large bumps spread on people; some were entirely covered. They spread everywhere, on the face, the head, the chest, etc.

> The pustules that covered people caused great desolation; very many people died of them.... The disease of pustules lasted a full sixty days.... And many were disabled and paralyzed by it. ...The Mexica warriors were greatly weakened by it. And when things were in this state, the Spaniards came.... (Lockhart 1993, 180–4)

In comparison, the Spanish text is very similar, yet shows important differences:

> Chapter twenty-nine, of the pestilence of smallpox that broke out among the Indians after the Spaniards left Mexico. But before the Spanish who were in Tlaxcala came to conquer Mexico, a pestilence of smallpox struck among all the Indians in the month they called Tepeihuitl, which is at the end of September. Very many Indians died of the pestilence; they had their whole bodies, faces, and limbs so full of pocks.... This pestilence killed innumerable people. ...The force of this pestilence lasted sixty days.... When this pestilence was ending in Mexico, the Spaniards ... arrived. (Lockhart 1993, 181–3)

Comparing both texts, it is striking that together, they produce the dichotomy of 'we' versus 'the Other.' While the Nahua text reports how "us," "the local people" and the "Mexica warriors" were affected by the illness, the Spanish text talks about the ill "Indians," introducing a common colonial classification of othering. The Nahuatl text sees no need to explain the name of the month of the Aztec calendar, but the Spanish text does; the Nahuatl version focuses on how the Mexica lived the illness, how it affected them. Meanwhile, the Spanish text also reports what the Spanish were doing at the time of the plague, privileging a European view. As the virus is Tenochtitlán's first European invader, followed by the conquerors, the Nahuatl text reflects on the value, restrictions, and alien control—all biopolitical measures—the ailment meant for them.

The conflict between biopolitical control and its resistance, constructed by the two text variants, continues throughout the Florentine Codex. As Sahagún and his team meticulously record the indigenous past and present, in book ten they also inform about Nahua doctors' work and about "los miembros de todo el cuerpo interiores y esteriores y de las enfermedades y medicinas contrarias [desta gente indiana]" (the interior and exterior body members and illnesses and medicines for remedy of these Indian people) (Sahagún 1577, iv). However, Sahagún also represents himself, the missionary, as a doctor of colonial 'spiritual illnesses' which he detects and uses medical language to metaphorize his work as a friar. Thus, he reflects the biopower over life and death proposed for Mexican people by his faith and religious institution:

El médico no puede acertadamente aplicar las medicinas al enfermo [sin] que primero, conozca de qué humor, o de qué causa procede la enfermedad; de manera que el buen médico conviene sea docto en el conocimiento de las medicinas y en el de las enfermedades, para aplicar convenientemente a cada enfermedad la medicina contraria y porque los predicadores y enfermos médicos son de las animas, para curar las enfermedades espirituales conviene que tengan experiencia de la medicina y de las enfermedades espirituales.

(A doctor cannot apply medication to the ill without knowing first from which humor the illness comes from and which causes it has; thus, a good doctor needs to be an expert in the knowledge of medicines and ailments, so to conveniently apply the medicine which counters each illness; and, as the preachers are healers of illnesses of the soul, they need to have experience in the spiritual medicine and ailments in order to cure spiritual illnesses). (Sahagún 1996, vol. 1, 24)

Sahagún repeats Galen's principles of internal body humors which cause illnesses and believes with Galen that contraries cure contraries, "contraria a contrariis curantur," which in sixteenth-century Europe was generally accepted medical knowledge. Even though his chronicles talk about the contagious spreading of smallpox, he ignores contemporary medical knowledge on external causes for physical suffering. At that time, thinkers like Girolamo Frascatore or Paracelsus have advanced a new understanding which would soon revolutionize medicine. Frascatore talks about extra-physical organisms—such as viral infections—attacking the body, and Paracelsus of the curing of illnesses with its own substance, which becomes the epistemological basis for vaccines.[4] By invoking his role as a "doctor of the soul" in the sense of Galen, Sahagún follows an acknowledged religious opinion of his time, privileging the spiritual health over the body's wellbeing (Worcester 2005; Sander 2014). At the same time, Sahagún replays the early modern biopolitical discourse which equates medicine and politics and metaphorizes both for each other: "If the organological metaphor is at the heart of political treatise, at the heart of the metaphor lies disease. ...[T]he point of intersection between political knowledge and medical knowledge is the common problem of preserving the body. ...[T]his preservation takes on a central role precisely from the perspective opened up by disease" (Esposito 2011, 121). While Sahagún's idea of the spiritual doctor represents European biomedical power over the colonized Other, his Codex Florentinus also undermines the very practice of othering, as it provides a space for this 'Other' to speak the 'Self.' A Nahua painting accompanies the Nahuatl description of the plague from 1520 (fig. 2), showing five affected people with pocks all over their skin. They are lying on woven mats and are covered with blankets. One of them is sitting in bed, and a doctor, the Nahua medical wise men *ticitl* (Boornazian Diel 2018, 59), is talking—the small curl-like figure before his face is the Nahua's sign for speech—and so is the ill person on the lower left side of the picture. Despite their condition, the Mexica are consciously speaking subjects for whom the contagious Other is necessarily the (viral) European invader.

---

4    All information on Galen and Paracelus are taken from Esposito (2011, 123–124), who analyses the shifting medical panorama in the sixteenth century from a biopolitical point of view and for a biopolitical theorizing.

*Figure 2:* Codex Florentinus *(ca. 1577), Biblioteca Medicea Laurenziana, Firenze (Sahagún 1577).*

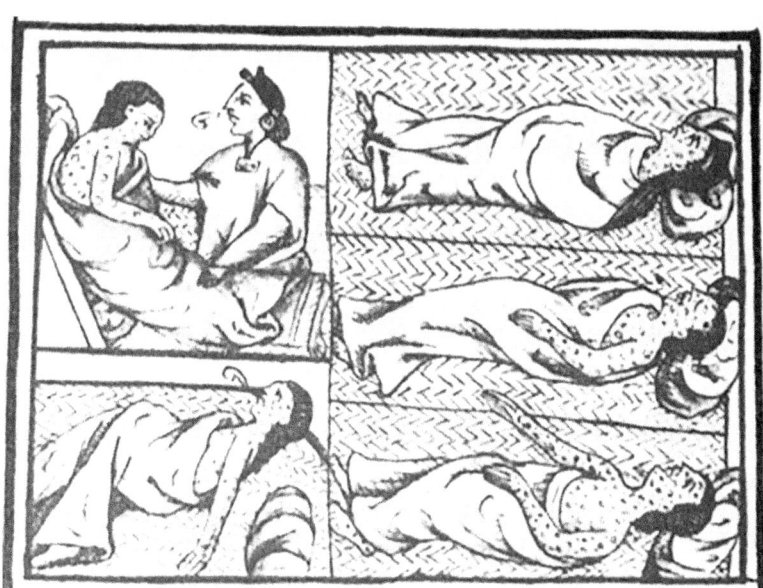

## Othering in COVID-19 Fictions

In COVID-19 fictions, the category of the Other, shaped by circumstances of coloniality and biopolitics, reappears. After the first wave of informal Corona literatures, popping up in large quantities on the internet in 2020, established authors in the Romance speaking world publish poetry, short narratives, and some novels in renowned editorials, especially from 2021 onwards.[5] This literary trend goes beyond the realist scope of the diaries and poems of the first quarantines,[6] and looks for alternative modes to express the concerns about the current pandemic. One example is Daniel Galera's *O deus das avencas* (*The*

---

5    "Covid-19"-novels from 2021 and 2022 are, for instance, Isabel Allende's novel *Violeta* (2022) or Miguel Sousa Tavares' *Ultimo olhar* (2021).

6    Poems like José Luís Peixotos *Regresso a casa* (2020), diaries like Gonçalo de Tavares *Diário da peste. O ano de 2020* (2021). For an overview of early COVID-19 literature in the Iberian Peninsula, see Grimaldi (2021).

*god of the maidenhair fern*), consisting of three short novels which take place in an uncertain future. In an interview from June 2021, the Brazilian author explains that he wrote the book during the pandemic, which greatly influenced his project:

> Comecei a novela ... antes da pandemia. ...Mas era como se aqueles meses ... já se situassem ... numa outra era geológica.... [N]ão podia prever ... a pandemia. Que talvez ressignifique toda a coisa do isolamento de Lucas e Manuela ... que se alonga indefinidamente.... E pra imaginar esse futuro tive de incorporar a realidade da pandemia e da nossa crise democrática ....

> (I started the short novel before the pandemic. ...But it was as if these months ... were already situated ... in another geological era. This is why, maybe, the whole thing of the isolation of Lucas and Manuela, which is indefinitely prolonged, took on a new meaning. ...And in order to imagine the future I had to incorporate the reality of the pandemic and of our democracy in crisis.) (Galera qtd. in Romanoff, 2021).

Galera's first short novel gives the volume its title and follows the isolation of a couple before the birth of their first child. The third short novel, *Bugônia*, circles around a pathogenic catastrophe. Galera, however, stresses that he imagined the story before the outbreak of Corona and that he did not change its figuration of the bacterium for the idea of the virus:

> Um sinal de que comecei a imaginar essas histórias antes da pandemia é que a ameaça patógena que assola os personagens são as famigeradas superbactérias resistentes. Evitei mudar isso depois que o vírus se tornou o emblema da morte que nos acompanha agora, pra que a ficção soasse como ficção.

> (One sign that I started to imagine these stories before the pandemic is that the pathogenic threat which devastates the characters are the notoriously resistant super bacteria. I avoided changing this after the virus transformed into the emblem of death which accompanies us now, so that the fiction would sound like fiction). (Galera qtd. in Romanoff, 2021)

In the second short novel, *Tóquio* [Tokyo], it becomes clear that the biopolitical space designed to life and death is now happening inside a privileged colony of the rich, while the exploited rest has to struggle for "bare" survival (Agamben 1998, 42, 97) outside the gated communities. The text presents a dystopic space—we are situated in a world shaped by pandemics, approximately in the 2050s, and builds on narratives which link hyper-technological development to distorted visions of the future (Aradau and Blanke 2022, 176–9). Such a world has apparently lost contact with its colonial Other:

> Aquela Tóquio seria desfigurada nas décadas seguintes pelo aquecimento do clima, pelas pandemias e pelas crises de abastecimento, se tornaria, como São Paulo e a maioria das megacidades, uma mistura de habitações improvisadas, fazendas urbanas e mercados de pulgas interligados por túneis desinfetados e refrigerados, cercada por vastidões de território inóspito e parcialmente demolido onde a luta pela sobrevivência ganhava feições que nós, os privilegiados que viviam no entorno das torres, tínhamos dificuldade para imaginar.

> (Tokyo would be disfigured in the following decades by global warming, the pandemics and supply crisis, and turned, like São Paulo and most megacities, into a mixture of improvised living spaces, urban farms and flee markets, interconnected by disinfected and air-conditioned tunnels, surrounded by a vastness of inhospitable, partly destroyed territory, where the struggle to survive took on proportions which we, the privileged inside the towers, could not even imagine). (Galera 2021, 72)

In Galera's post- and pluripandemic world, the (poor, racialized, colonized) Other is, on one hand, eliminated from the depicted Brazilian society, but it reappears, on the other hand, in the form of androids, human beings who once stored their brains on hard drives and who are now, due to the shortage of raw material and financial crisis, an inconvenient asset to contemporary society. In a meeting with a hyperrealist android, the narrator feels "atravessado por uma descarga de desejo sexual" (crossed by a discharge of sexual desire) (Galera 2021, 51), and shortly after, by a wave of shame, as if he was reproducing what Frantz Fanon described as the desire for the colonized Other: "Face to face with this man who is 'different from himself,' he needs ... to personify The Other. The Other will become the mainstay of his preoccupations and his desires" ([1952] 2008, 131). As Galera's short novel asks—but never answers—what to do with the new army of technologized Others, who cannot longer be repaired and whom nobody wants to be responsible for, the—unrepairable—Brazilian colonial past comes to mind, and the avoidance of taking responsibility for ongoing exclusion, violence and colonial trauma (Rothberg 2008, Andermahr 2015).

Alongside shorter narrations on COVID-19 like Galera's, Valter Hugo Mãe's lyrical novel *As Doenças do Brasil* (*Brasil's Illnesses*) was published in Portugal in 2021. Even though the novel does not mention the current pandemic with any word, it is hard not to read this text on illness through the lens of COVID-19 fictions. Contrary to Galera's futurist visions, Mãe turns to the past and places the story in colonial Brazil. Mãe's prose plays with a perspective which apparently comes from within a native Brazilian community, the Abaeté. The polyphone, poetic language tries to disrupt nostalgically appropriating visions towards the indigenous Other. Mãe invents a "uma narrativa estranha, que … desorientará a leitura" (a narrative of strangeness which disorients reading) through a "cruzamento de sintaxe tupi e portuguesa, ou melhor, enxerta na língua portuguesa atual a mundivisão tupi" (crossing of Tupi and Portguese sintaxis, or more precisely, he inserts the Tupi world vision into the Portuguese language) (Real 2021). Even if the insertion of Tupi thinking into the colonizer's language must remain a literary construct, the approach to native cosmovision translates, for instance, in conversations which end in "Não sinto" (I don't feel), as for "I don't understand" (Mãe 2021, 71).

The Angolese-Portuguese author Mãe dedicates the novel to Ailton Krenak, one of Brazil's most prominent native intellectuals, writers, and activists, who publicly denounced Brazil's governmental necropolitics during COVID-19, recalling the societal and epidemiological risks of contact and contagion which Western culture has always meant for indigenous peoples:

> [O]s epidemologistas … estão dizendo que o evento do covid é resultado da nossa promiscuidade. …Nós estamos fazendo uma política de morte ao invés de estarmos fazendo uma política de vida. …[T]emos uma decisão clara do Estado brasilero de … assolar a vida indígena, e uma pandemia. …E a violência garimpeira, a violência madeireira … [n]os territórios indígenas, o assassinato, … e um contágio em cima.

> (Epidemologists say that the event of Covid is the result of our promiscuity…. We produce a politics of death instead of a politics of life. We have a clear decision from the Brazilian State to attack indigenous life, and a pandemic. …And the violence of diamond extraction and the wood industry in indigenous territories, murder, … moreover, contagion). (Krenak 2020, 27–35)

As Krenak's points to practices of biopolitical othering during COVID-19 and connects them to the colonial past, Mãe's novel resumes that colonial acts have always been the true illness of Brazil. As leading motto of his novel, Mãe places various excerpts of colonial Portuguese writing, most prominently a sermon by António Vieira from 1638 which analyzes "[a] causa original das doenças do Brasil: tomar o alheio, cobiças, interesses, ganhos" (the original cause of Brazil's illness: taking from the other, avarice, interests, profit) (Vieira qtd. in Mãe 2021, 10). Once more, Vieira metaphorizes the ill body to express the (bio)political malaise of colonial societies and the deteriorated "health of the State" (Esposito 2011, 121), on the basis of Galen's humoral theory:

> E como tantos sintomas lhe sobrevêm ao pobre enfermo, e todos acometem à cabeça e ao coração, que são as partes mais vitais, e todos dão atrativos e contrativos do dinheiro, que é o nervo … das repúblicas, fica tomado todo o corpo, e tolhido de pés e mãos, sem haver mão esquerda que castigue, nem mão direita que premie, e, faltando a justiça punitiva para explelir os humores nocivos, … milagre é que não tenha expirado.

> (And so many symptoms overcome the poor sick, and they all attack head and heart, the most vital parts, and all tempt and contract money, which is the nerve of republics, so that the whole body ends up infested, with disabled feet and hands, without a left hand to punish or a right hand to award, and, as the punitive justice to expel the harmful humors is missing …, it is a wonder that the body has not yet expired). (Vieira qtd. in Mãe 2021, 11).

The poor health of the colonized—Other—"social body" (Foucault 1976, 192), which Vieira describes, suffers due to the imperial condition which violates Brazil's people. Mãe's novel centers around the character Honra (Honor), who forms part of the remote Abaté community, where he represents the Other: his Abaté mother was raped and Honra is the son of a European. In the logics of the village, the colonial order represents illness. One day, the communities' pajé, or shaman, announces that Honra's role is to help to understand this 'white plague,' "E conheci que ele será ensinado na língua inimiga do branco para ser mascarado de branco e trazer à nosse comunidade a informação sobre a multiplicação dessa malignidade." (And I learned that he will be taught the enemy language of the white to be disguised as white and to bring information about the multiplication of this malignancy) (Mãe 2021, 73). The invaders appear as cancerous tumor, as infectious illness, and while Honra is contemplating his role of the Other in his community, he dreams of healing from what he calls his 'white wound.' "Honra pensava que se a nova era houvesse de chegar lhe curaria a cor e o sangue" (Honra thought that if the new era would come, it would heal his color and blood) (Mãe 2021, 64). Honra's desire to stop being the (contagious) Other reflects once more the colonized "desire to be suddenly *white*," which is hidden in the "blackest part of my soul, across the zebra striping of my mind" (Fanon [1952] 2008, 45, italics in original). Reflecting on imperial administration and disease control and published during the COVID pandemic, the novel *As doenças do Brasil* might be *the* great allegory for the biopolitical coloniality of illness.

## Conclusions

What do two bodies of text have in common when they are as diverse as the one formed by sixteenth-century colonial literature and the other consisting of contemporary COVID-19 fiction? And moreover, are these bodies of texts not fragmented within themselves? The analysis of this article started out with one of the probably best-known Spanish chronicles of the conquest of America, Bernal Díaz del Castillo's *Historia verdadera*, only to combine it with the structurally and culturally diverse format which the Florentine Codex offers. While the first one produces the contagious Other, the viral scape goat, in the figuration of the African slave—a victim of colonial biopolitics—the Florentine Codex' bilingual character stays undecided whether to support or resist colonial biopolitics, and thus, engages in both. As the Spanish part of the text constructs the sick Other, the pustule-covered Indian, the Nahuatl version powerfully defends 'us, the people' who collectively endure and fight colonial (viral) invasion. The picture of the speaking Self, the Nahua doctor, and his patients, is more than a mere illustration, but stands up for their right to live in the face of textual strategies of othering.

The article then jumped 500 years ahead to scenarios of coloniality and its practices of biopolitical othering in current COVID-19 fictions. Daniel Galera's short novel *Tóquio*, produced under the influence of the pandemic, imagines a dystopic future in which the colonial Other has become unrecognizable, yet remains structurally present, as disposable, human-like android creating sexual desire. This article also read Valter Hugo Mãe's *As doenças do Brasil*—a novel which not once mentions COVID-19—as *the* allegory of biopolitical functioning of coloniality during viral infections. Written and published during the Corona pandemic, *As doenças do Brasil* builds on a seventeenth-century 'biopolitical' sermon by Padre Vieira about the ill condition of the colonized social body. Mãe invents a poetic language which seeks to deconstruct and reconstruct the contagious Other, no longer in the figure of the indisposed subalternalized, but in the idea of colonial biopolitics' evil operations.

These two parts of the article's text corpus are fragmented within themselves, and they do not obey the borders of history or genre: a "non-COVID" COVID-fiction, *As doenças do Brasil*, accompanies a dystopia, *Tóquio*, in which colonial structures are vaguely recognizable; a hybrid text, the Florentine Codex, clashes against itself and against the straight, but imaginary rich narrative of authenticity presented by Bernal Díaz del Castillo. And yet, this article suggests a continuity of language, symbols and practices which act across the frontiers of time and text convention, portraying domination through the evaluation and measurement of the physical, and constructing or questioning the value, disposability, restriction, and control over the (post)colonial Other. Together, the analyzed texts depict biopolitical conditions favoring infection and death, the technological or military procedures which deepen society's gaps and produce the sick Other. Both parts of the text corpus establish a narrative of immediacy. The horror of illness and death has no present nor future but exists as an ever-present warning. The gaze onto the ill body of the Other tells discrepant stories, depending on the position of the speaker. COVID-Fictions about the Other talk back to imperial agents and notions; in the Florentine codex's image, the ill Mexica with their graphically archived voices have the power to speak. They also remind us, in the words of Julia Kristeva, that the Other is us, and that we are the Other ([1988] 1990, 208–9), and that concepts of the Self and the Other are, once more, reconstructed in viral times.

## Works Cited

Adorno, Rolena. 1988. "El sujeto colonial y la construcción de la alteridad." *Revista de Crítica Literaria Latinoamericana* 14, no. 28: 55–68.

Agamben, Giorgio. 1998. *Homo Sacer: Sovereign Power and Bare Life*. Translated by Daniel Heller-Roazen. Stanford: Stanford University Press.

Alencar Jr., Osmar G. 2020. "Crise global e a necropolítica do governo Bolsonaro em tempos de pandemia." *Ciências Sociais Unisonos* 56, no. 3: 266–76.

Andermahr, Sonya. 2015. "Decolonizing Trauma Studies: Trauma and Postcolonialism." *Humanities* 4, no. 4: 500–5.

Aradau, Claudia, and Tobias Blanke. 2022. *Algorithmic Reason: The New Government of Self and Other*. Oxford: Oxford University Press.

Boornazian Diel, Lori. 2018. *The Codex Mexicanus: A Guide to Life in Late-Sixteenth Century New Spain*. Austin: University of Texas Press.

Bragato, Fernanda F., Marco A. Delfino de Almeida, and Jocelyn G. Kestenbaum. 2020. "Povos Indígenas, Genocídio e Pademia No Brasil." *Revista Culturas Jurídicas* 7, no. 17: 80–109.

Brooks, Francis. 2003. "The Impact of Disease." In *Technology, Disease, and Colonial Conquests Sixteenth to Eighteenth Centuries: Essays Reappraising the Guns and Germs Theories*, edited by George Raudenz, 127–65. Boston: Brill.

Butler, Judith. 2020. "Capitalism Has Its Limits." *Verso* (blog). March 30, 2020. https://www.versobooks.com/blogs/4603-capitalism-has-its-limits.

Caponi, Sandra. 2021. "Biopolitica, necropolítica e racismo na gestão de Covid-19." *Revista Porto das Letras* 7, no. 2: 22–44.

Chervenski Figueira, Guillerme, Pedro Bambil Souza, Sandra Cristina de Souza, and Joseph Calabres. 2020. "Povos Indígenas e a pandemia Covid 19 no Brasil, um genocídio anunciado." *Ipê Roxo* 2, no. 1: 95–110.

Christ, Gui. 2020. *The Luxury of Social Isolation*. https://guichrist.com/portfolio/commisions/paraisopolis/.

Crosby, Alfred W. (1986) 2015. *Ecological Imperialism: The Biological Expansion of Europe, 900–1900*. Austin: University of Texas Press.

De Sousa Santos, Boaventura. 2020. *La cruel pedagogía del virus*. Translated by Paula Vasile. Ciudad Autónoma de Buenos Aires: CLACSO.

Díaz del Castillo, Bernal. 2015. *Historia verdadera de la conquista de la Nueva España*. Edited by Guillermo Seres. Madrid: Real Academia Española.

"Los ecos de la caída de Tenochtitlan 500 años después." *El País*, August 13, 2021. https://elpais.com/mexico/2021-08-13/los-ecos-de-la-caida-de-tenochtitlan-500-anos-despues.html.

Esposito, Roberto. 2011. *Immunitas: The Protection and Negation of Life*. Translated by Zakiya Hanafi. Cambridge: Polity.

Fanon, Frantz. (1952) 2008. *Black Skin, White Masks*. Translated by Charles Lam Markmann. London: Pluto Press.

Favrot Peterson, Jeanette. 2019. "Images in Translation: A Codex 'Muy Historiado.'" In *The Florentine Codex: An Encyclopedia of the Nahua World in Sixteenth-Century Mexico*, edited by Jeanette Favrot Peterson and Kevin Terraciano, 21–36. Austin: University of Texas Press.

Ferreira, Ricardo Bruno Santos, and Climene Laura de Camargo. 2021. "Vulnerabilidade da população negra brasileira frente à evolução da pandemia por COVID-19." *Revista Cuidarte* 12, no. 2: 1–12.

Foucault, Michel. 1976. *Histoire de la sexualité I: La volonté de savoir*. Paris: Gallimard.

———. (1997) 2003. "Society Must Be Defended." In *Lectures at the Collège de France 1975–1976*, translated by David Macey. Picador: New York.

Galera, Daniel. 2021. *O deus das avencas: Três novelas*. São Paulo: Companhia das Letras.

Grimaldi, Susanne. 2021. "'Este presente de remolino.' La primera primavera pandémica en la Península Ibérica." *Estudios Culturales Hispánicos* 2: 155–96.

Jáuregui, Carlos A., and David Solodkow. 2019. "Biopolitics and the Farming (of) Life in Bartolomé de las Casas." *Studies in the History of Christian Traditions* 189: 127–66.

Krenak, Ailton. 2020. *A vida não é útil*. São Paulo: Companhia das Letras.

Kristeva, Julia. (1988) 1990. *Fremde sind wir uns selbst*. Translated by Xenia Rajewsky. Frankfurt a. M.: Suhrkamp.

Lockhart, James. 1993. Introduction to *We People Here: Nahuatl Accounts of the Conquest of Mexico*, translated and edited by James Lockhart, 1–46. Berkeley: University of California Press.

Mãe, Valter Hugo. 2021. *As doenças do Brasil*. Porto: Porto Editora.

Malvido, Elsa, and Carlos Viesca. 1985. "La epidemia de cocoliztli de 1576." *Historias* 11: 24–33.

Martínez del Río de Redo, Marita. 2005. "Una Visión Singular De La Conquista De México." In *Imágenes De Los Naturales En El Arte De La Nueva España Siglos XVI Al XVIII*, edited by Elisa Vargas Lugo de Bosch, 124–135. Mexico City: Fomento Cultural Banamex.

Mbembe, Joseph-Achille. 2003. "Necropolitics." Translated by Libby Meintjes. *Public Culture* 15, no. 1: 11–40.

Pereira Campos dos Santos, Herbert Luan, Fernanda Beatriz Melo Maciel, Kênia Rocha Santos, Cídia Dayara Vieira Silva da Conceição, Rian Silva de Oliveira, Natiene Ramos Ferreira da Silva, and Nília Maria de Brito Lima Prado. 2020. "Necropolítica e reflexões acerca da população negra no contexto da pandemia da COVID-19 no Brasil: uma revisão bibliográfica." *Ciência e Saúde Coletiva* 25, no. 2: 4211–24.

Quijano, Aníbal. 2014. "Colonialidad del poder, eurocentrismo y América Latina." In *Cuestiones y horizontes: Antología esencial: De la dependencia histórico-estructural a la colonialidad/descolonialidad del poder*, edited by Danilo Assis Clímaco, 777–832. Buenos Aires: CLACSO.

Rao, Ida Giovanna. 2019. "On the Reception of the Florentine Codex: The First Italian Translation." In *The Florentine Codex: An Encyclopedia of the Nahua*

*World in Sixteenth-Century Mexico*, edited by Jeanette Favrot Peterson and Kevin Terraciano, 37–44. Austin: University of Texas Press.

Real, Miguel. 2021. "Valter Hugo Mãe—Um romance notável." *Jornal de Letras*. October 21, 2021. https://visao.sapo.pt/jornaldeletras/2021-10-20-valter-h ugo-mae-um-romance-notavel/.

Romanoff, Ricardo. 2021. "Daniel Galera explora futuros distópicos em 'O Deus das Avencas.'" *Matinal Jornalismo*. June 24, 2021. https://www.matinaljorna lismo.com.br/rogerlerina/literatura/o-deus-das-avencas-daniel-galera/.

Rothberg, Michael. 2008. "Decolonizing Trauma Studies: A Response." *Studies in the Novel* 40, no. 1/2: 224–34.

Safatle, Vladimir. 2021. "Para além da necropolítica." *N-1 Edições*. https://www. n-1edicoes.org/textos/191.

Sahagún, Bernardino de. 1577. "The Florentine Codex. Book X: The People, Their Virtues and Vices, and Other Nations." *Library of Congress*. https://www.loc .gov/item/2021667855.

———. 1996. *Historia general de las cosas de la Nueva España*. Edited by Alfredo López Austin and Guadalupe Quintana. México: Alianza Editorial Mexicana.

Sander, Christoph. 2014. "Medical Topics in the De anima Commentary of Coimbra (1598) and the Jesuits' Attitude towards Medicine in Education and Natural Philosophy." *Early Science and Medicine* 19, no. 1: 76–101.

Silva, Marcelo, and Elaine Cristina Francisco Volpato. 2020. "Trabalho Escravo Contemporâneo e a Pandemia SARS-COV-2: Reflexões sobre o Biopoder, a Biopolítica e a Necropolítica." *Cadernos de Dereito Actual* 14: 256–76.

Spagnesi, Enrico. 1993. "Bernardino de Sahagún, la natura in Messico, l'arte a Firenze." *Quaderni di Neotropica* 1: 7–24.

Spivak, Gayatri Chakravorty. 1994. "Can the Subaltern Speak?" In *Colonial Discourse and Post-Colonial Theory: A Reader*, edited by Laura Chrisman and Patrick Williams, 82–3. New York: Columbia University Press.

Terraciano, Kevin. 2019. "Introduction: An Encyclopedia of Nahua Culture; Context and Content." In *The Florentine Codex: An Encyclopedia of the Nahua World in Sixteenth-Century Mexico*, edited by Jeanette Favrot Peterson and Kevin Terraciano, 1–18. Austin: University of Texas Press.

Todorov, Tzvetan. (1982) 1999. *The Conquest of America: The Question of the Other*. Translated by Richard Howard. Norman: University of Oklahoma Press.

Tommaselli, Guilherme. 2020. "Necropolítica, Racismo e Governo Bolsonaro." *Caderno Prudentino de Geografia* 4, no. 42: 179–99.

Townsend, Camilla. 2017. *Annals of Native America: How the Nahuas of Colonial Mexico Kept Their History Alive*. Oxford: Oxford University Press.

Vainfas, Ronaldo. 2020. "A peste das Bexigas no Brasil colonial: tragédia histórica ou genocídio?" *Brathair* 20, no. 2: 107–27.

Worcester, Thomas. 2005. "A Defensive Discourse: Jesuits on Disease in Seventeenth-Century New France." *French Colonial History* 6: 1–15.

# 3. 'Enlightened' Colonialism, Smallpox, and the Indigenous Other in Late Eighteenth-Century Mexico and Guatemala

*Martin Gabriel*

During the colonial era, different epidemics regularly devastated many areas of Spain's American Empire. Influenza, measles or smallpox killed millions, most of them indigenous people. This contribution will focus on the outbreaks of, reactions to, and countermeasures against smallpox in Guatemala and Oaxaca (Mexico) in 1780 and 1796/97, respectively. While both areas might not be representative of Spanish America in general, they are well-suited for research focusing on processes of 'othering' in a colonial context because of their unusually large indigenous populations. In this chapter, I will explore the prevalence of smallpox in Spanish American history, the state-run smallpox response during the outbreaks in Guatemala and Oaxaca in the late eighteenth century, and the processes of racialization and ethnic stratification of society in this context. Indigenous subjects of the Spanish crown were often seen as ambivalent: on the one hand, they were characterized as docile and childlike persons in need of paternalistic support, on the other hand, administrators and clerics feared widespread idolatry and rebellion, and thus were interested in bringing more Amerindians under efficient imperial control (Chuchiak 2005, 645; Clendinnen 1982, 43). Spanish anti-smallpox strategies in Guatemala, Oaxaca, and other regions of the empire illustrate the ambivalence of eighteenth-century political, social or intellectual 'reform' with countermeasures existing in an intermediate stage between traditional, early modern (or medieval) European strategies and new protective measures that would only leave their imprint from the early 1800s on. However, anti-contagion measures can be defined as part of a larger framework of 'modernist' and 'reformist' ideas that were central to many aspects of imperial policy during the Bourbon era (Gabriel 2019).

Since the human immune system's efficiency "hinges on the ability to distinguish self from non-self" (Jones 2003, 725), infectious diseases are per se connected to the question of Otherness. Like the coronavirus (COVID-19) pandemic in the twenty-first century, infectious diseases in early modern colonial environments were often discursively tied to a more or less clearly specified Other. "Defining the Other comes to attribute a different status—juridical, cultural, and social—than the majority" or the group dominating official discourses (Kastoryano 2010, 81). In the case of COVID-19, long-standing tropes of animosity and racism towards China and people of Chinese origin were prevalent especially during the earlier months of the crisis (Moynihan and Porumbescu 2020). During disease outbreaks in colonial Spanish America, identifying certain social or ethnic groups as 'super spreaders,' as immune or especially vulnerable often created social, ethnic or other divisions, while, at the same time, in many cases it continued to reproduce already existing models of differentiation. A typical trope focused on indigenous peoples dying by the thousands from an infectious disease, while Europeans in the same area did not succumb to the sickness. Of course, these discourses were not 'neutral,' but implied specific assumptions about hygiene or physical resilience of the colonial Other; only through the creation of 'othered' groups "could the introduction of the motto 'knowledge is power' enter in the development of modern identity" (Kaya 2018, 177; Motolinía 1971, 30). As with COVID-19, there was no immediate master plan to respond to the crises, and different measures (travel bans, quarantines, inoculation, etc.) implemented by state administrators led to different reactions of the populace, ranging from widespread support to physical violence.

The eighteenth-century smallpox (*variola*) epidemics in Guatemala and Oaxaca did not come as a surprise. The Americas had, most likely, been in contact with this disease since Columbus's second fleet—that transported also colonists and friars—had arrived from Cádiz in the autumn of 1493. Catholic clergymen reported an outbreak on Hispaniola in 1518/19 (Cook 2002, 363–7; Rigau-Pérez 1982, 424). The main reasons for this chronological delay might have been the introduction of the less fatal *variola minor* prior to the deadly *variola maior* strain as well as the fact that it was almost exclusively adult males who "went to the Caribbean in the earliest decades of contact, which automatically excluded non-immune or infectious individuals. With a voyage of six weeks or more, an individual who had acquired smallpox in Europe would have...either died or become immune and non-infectious by the time he reached the Americas" (Curtin 1993, 350–1).

Smallpox is caused by an orthopox virus and relies solely on human victims as carriers (Brooks 1993, 12); protracted close contact between persons is of enormous relevance for spreading the disease (Riley 2010, 454–5). Case-fatality rates for *variola minor* have been set at around only one percent, while those for *variola maior*, even after the introduction of the Jennerian smallpox vaccine, remained stable at above 20 percent (Carmichael and Silverstein 1987, 149). Typical symptoms of smallpox infections were a rash, fever, vomiting, mucocutaneous hemorrhages as well as corneal infections that left victims permanently blind (Barquet and Domingo 1997, 636). Alfred Crosby's idea of "virgin soil epidemics" spreading among peoples never confronted with a specific pathogen before has been criticized for not considering "evidence that American Indians were no more susceptible...than other populations where the diseases had not struck within the lifetime of the people" (Newman 1976, 671). Immunological memory and adaptive immunity—or its absence—played an important role in the spreading of epidemiological diseases; however, factors such as population density, diet, genetics or co-infections with other diseases resulted in a great variety of actual infection patterns (Ramenofsky, Wilbur, and Stone 2003, 251). Malnutrition, for example, has been recognized as "most common cause of secondary immunodeficiency in the world" (Sandberg, Kline, and Shearer 1996, 565); some researchers focusing on smallpox, however, have instead underlined the negative effects of "social disruption" (such as lack of nursing) during *variola* outbreaks (Riley 2010, 457–61).

## European Invasion and Demographic Crisis in New Spain

There is little doubt that smallpox was introduced into what is now Mexico in the first half of 1520 at the latest. While some authors suggest a depopulation of central Mexico already beginning in 1518, sustained Euro-Mexican cultural contact did not exist at that time and many details remain unclear (Jones 2014, 497; Riley 2010, 450). In August of 1520, Lucas Vázquez de Ayllón reported to King Carlos I that he had encountered indigenous inhabitants of Cozumel Island (off Yucatán) who had obviously been infected with smallpox; he reasoned that the disease had been introduced by Pánfilo de Narváez's expeditionary force a few months earlier (McCaa 1995, 402). If "patient zero" was indeed a man of African descent is impossible to verify—nonetheless, it is telling to see a man marked as non-European Other being identified as the person responsible for the epidemic (Behbehani 1983, 458; Brooks 1993, 19). This speaks to the long-standing tradition of blaming 'outsiders' for diseases and helps to clear Europeans of the responsibility for the devastation of indigenous societies; on the other hand, however, the African man could be seen as instrumental in the conquest of the Americas—not as a scapegoat, but as important figure in God's plan for the expansion of Christendom.

After the horrific sixteenth-century epidemics, New Spain had lost a large percentage of its original population. However, demographic decline did not simply result from 'natural' events like diseases; the origins of population losses were also to be found in the sociopolitical realities and factors such as excessive labor requirements (Jones 2003, 705; Moreno Okuno and Ventosa-Santaulària 2010, 94). Inhumane working conditions, for example, contributed to the spread of disease and increased mortality among infected populations. The history of epidemics in Spanish America hence needs to take into account European perspectives on othered (primarily indigenous) populations who could be subjugated and their labor extracted as part of colonial rule (Livi-Bacci 2006, 204; López de Mariscal 2008, 79). Arguments focusing solely on the aspect of infection and on indigenous bodies as "soft fodder for aggressive Old World pathogens" (Hämäläinen 2010, 174) will fall short.

Horrific losses notwithstanding, Amerindian peoples did not disappear. Population recovery in the Americas turned out to be dependent on specific regional circumstances: in Yucatán, this process began in the first half of the seventeenth century, while the region of the Isthmus of Tehuantepec (the geographical border of North and Central America) experienced a demographic decline until the beginning of the eighteenth century (Díaz-Polanco and Burguete 1989, 100; Few 2012, 303). While there might have been fewer supra-regional epidemics once smaller populations could not sustain "reservoirs" of non-immune hosts, outbreaks of non-endemic infectious diseases are often known to be much more devastating (Jones 2003, 732; Riley 2010, 477; Thompson 2018, 141).

Turning our attention to Guatemala, it becomes obvious that this region was hit hard by a number of different infectious diseases already during the early phase of the *conquista*. Between 1520 (four years prior to Pedro de Alvarado's campaign of conquest) and 1632, at least eight supra-regional and about two dozen local or regional outbreaks of epidemics such as measles, smallpox or bubonic plague devastated the region (Lovell 1992, 434; Lovell 1988, 29; Veblen 1977, 490). Diseases, combined with violence, displacement, and famines, continued to hamper economic development, resulting in lower tax revenues, less incentives to invest in Guatemala, and fewer possibilities to deal with crises (such as epidemics) when they arose. Only at the end of the eighteenth century, a large-scale export economy, based on indigo, developed; however, plantations were concentrated in the south, not the peripheral Mayan regions in the north (Megged 1992, 437; Palma Murga 2007, 102; Tedlock 1993, 141–2). As late as the 1760s, Spaniards were framed as Other by Maya in times of political conflict: during the "Quisteil Rebellion" of 1761, indigenous fighters were encouraged to kill pigs whose eradication would, allegedly, lead to the death of Spaniards as well (Pugh 2009, 376). It is well known that, for example, in sixteenth-century Mexico, the behavior of Franciscans was so foreign to local people that they othered the Europeans in an extreme way: they characterized them as sick, senseless, mad, and doomed to die (Muñoz Camargo 1966, 166); obviously, such approaches had not totally disappeared by the late 1700s. For Spaniards, this demonstrated the need to integrate non-European populations into the colonial framework; health policies could foster this integration since they related not only to medical issues, but also cultural and religious worldviews. Colonial policies remained ambivalent: the hierarchization of society depended on framing many (not all) Amerindians as Other, while, at the same time, officials aimed at integrating these othered groups more efficiently into the realm. Inoculation programs directed exclusively at indigenous people were among the most important strategies. In some sense, these activities were 'humanist', but they were also based on the identification of the colonized Other (Few 2012). We also have to keep in mind that there was an ethno-social divide between the people responsible for fighting epidemics and the majority of the population: at least in theory, physicians had to prove 'pure' Spanish ancestry (*limpieza de sangre*) before being certified by the medical governing board, the *Protomedicato* (Hernández Sáenz 2000, 35–6).

## The 1780 Smallpox Outbreak in Guatemala

At the beginning of the 1780s, the practice of inoculation had already been implemented in different regions of the Spanish Empire such as Chile, Peru or Mexico City, where a smallpox epidemic had killed about 9,000 inhabitants in the "autumn of death" (*otoño de la muerte*) of 1779 (Mark and Rigau-Pérez 2009, 66; Miño Grijalva 2012, 602; Smith 1974, 10). The eighteenth century saw inoculation or variolation campaigns being implemented by many European states; however, the tradition of inoculating against smallpox had been known centuries earlier in China. During inoculation, infected material was taken from

pustules or scabs and introduced through cuts in a person's skin or via the
nasal tract (Bazin 2000, 9; Janssens 1981, 250). Inoculation notwithstanding, in
most areas under European rule, isolation, quarantines or trade prohibitions
were generally seen as the most efficient defensive measures against smallpox
(Smith 1974, 10; Thompson 1993, 432). After an earthquake seven years earlier,
Guatemalan authorities, in 1780, were still in the process of moving the capital
to Nueva Guatemala; Martha Few identified this fact as being of central importance because "institutions and cultures were in flux, opening space for trying
a new (Guatemalan) smallpox response" (2010, 523). Notably, there had been
widespread unrest among Guatemala's Maya after the 1773 earthquake, and ru-
mors about a new indigenous "king" also responsible for the capital's destruction had spread through Highland communities (Frühsorge 2011, 93). Again,
this (geological and social) instability served as a reminder for Spaniards to
find a solution for dealing with indigenous groups who were seen as royal subjects, but also as potential rebels trying to overthrow the political order. The
1780 inoculation campaign led by José Flores proved to be a veritable success
since mortality rates among inoculated persons were low; the introduction of
inoculation into the Kingdom of Guatemala was seen as proof of the benefi-
cial effects of European-style medical sciences (Few 2012, 312–3; Secretaría de
Estado 1796c, 1r–2r; Smith 1974, 10–1). Measures like inoculating colonial subjects during the eighteenth century have to be seen in the context of a 'modernization' discourse and ideas of more 'efficient' rule. Thus, internal stability,
effective evangelization, and the promotion of indigenous peoples' self-iden-
tification as colonial *subjects* can be seen as some of the "derivative functions of
medicine" (De Burgos 2014, 401). Spanish revenues primarily originated from
trade and production—a healthy workforce was paramount for both, and in
regions like Chiapas (then a part of the *audiencia* of Guatemala), profitability,
in the absence of important natural resources, rested primarily on population
numbers and what Carlos Jáuregui and David Solodkow have called the "systemic instrumentalization of life" (2018, 132; Ramírez 2012, 204; Viqueira 1994,
240–1). For much of the colonial era, a majority of medical practitioners in
Spain or its dependencies were healers, barber-surgeons or clerics rather than
academics and, while the latter were often scornful of "folk" practitioners, European-style treatments in many cases turned out to be useless (De Bevoise
1990, 153–4; Few 2018, 169; Newson 2006, 371–3). On the other hand, European physicians regularly included pre-Columbian knowledge when dealing
with illness (Foster 1987, 363; Fredrick 2021), not only in the colonial core regions like Central Mexico, but even more so on the edges of the empire, where

practitioners had "to look to the people and the earth around them for cures" (Crocker 2014, 298). In contemporary Maya communities, ritual specialists still perform a variety of duties such as healers, bonesetters, herbalists or astrologists (Hinojosa 2002, 28–32; Mayer 2015, 107; Pitarch 2007, 195). In rural parts of Oaxaca, approaches such as 'ethno-obstetrics'—applied mostly by indigenous midwives—continue to play an important role in everyday life. While researchers have long focused on the socioreligious or even magical elements of 'folk' healing (thus continuing the othering of indigenous traditions), modern surveys have pointed out its empirical underpinnings (Eliade 1951; Sesia 1996; Waldstein and Adams 2006, 105).

In the eighteenth century, policies related to topics like public hygiene, sanitation or anti-contagion measures were closely intertwined with issues of state control, and colonial elites, administrators, military leaders, and physicians characterized medical humanitarianism as a means of integrating multi-ethnic populations (Few 2012, 316). While anti-smallpox activities in 1780 were deemed a success, more than 10,000 indigenous inhabitants of the *audiencia* of Guatemala perished; in many cases, simply because protective measures or inoculation could not be applied in remote settlements. Sharonah Fredrick recently identified abundant water supplies and traditions of cleanliness as the reason why "the Mayan and the Andean peoples did not die in numbers as great as those of Aztecs or Europeans from smallpox, malaria, measles, and plague" (2021, 166), however, historical realities were much more complicated. The Mayan settlement of Bachajon in Chiapas reported more deaths in 1780 than in the years from 1772 through 1779 and from 1781 through 1794 combined; more than 4,400 people died in the remote Cuchumatán Highlands, almost 60 percent of the victims were children or youths (Andrieu 2010, 256; Lovell 2021, 21; Montero Lazcano 2020, 42–3). The colonial state, however, thought of its measures against smallpox as victory: population losses were reduced as can be seen from official statements on death rates among inoculated and non-inoculated people, and (maybe even more importantly) surviving indigenous populations could now be integrated into the Spanish administrative framework more efficiently, for the inoculation campaign was closely linked to a more permanent presence of state officials (Secretaría de Estado 1796c: 1r–2r). Inoculation campaigns such as those in Guatemala were "among the first areas in which the State's power was applied directly and tangibly" (Baldwin 1999, 245). This strategy was also obvious in the survey of Guatemalan lands; in that case, however, the top-down approach seems to have been more diluted and decisions relied much more on debate and negotiation (Hill 1989, 175–7; Sampeck 2014, 176). An unsuccessful example of forced integration was the removal of images of Catholic saints from the care of indigenous sodalities (*cofradías*) as part of "anti-idolatry campaigns" in 1799 (Orellana 1981, 170). Again, the state tried to force specific groups to give up traditional rights, but was unable to go through with its top-down policies.

Mayan communities, unlike those of Africans or *castas* (the offspring of mothers and fathers of different ethnic classification), were provided medical and organizational support during the epidemic—however, indigenous people had to take part in the funding of anti-contagion activities by payments from their community chests (Few 2010, 526–7). This shows the importance of Mayan groups for the imperial project: while many Mayans lived at the fringes of imperial control, state and church officials were interested in them as a potential workforce, but also as believers in Christianity; the ideas of economic stability of the empire, European 'enlightenment', and Catholic missionization converged in the administrative region of Guatemala.

Focusing countermeasures on the indigenous populace made sense from a demographic point of view, since *indios* and *indias* constituted the majority of Guatemala's inhabitants. This specific approach also shows that race and ethnicity played a central role in the colonial administration's response to smallpox in 1780. Unlike yellow fever that killed scores of Spaniards in Yucatán and thousands of British or French soldiers during campaigns in the Caribbean in the seventeenth and eighteenth centuries, smallpox was identified as a disease of indigenous populations (McNeill 1999, 179–80; Patch 1996, 734). Introducing smallpox inoculation, sending administrators to peripheral regions, and making indigenous communities pay for services definitely constituted the application of structural force towards a colonial Other in need of paternalistic control and support that, in the self-imagination of the colonial state, could only be provided by Europeans.

## Smallpox in the Intendancy of Oaxaca (1796/97)

Spanish anti-contagion measures against the smallpox epidemic of 1796/97 also have to be seen against the backdrop of the Bourbon dynasty's paternalistic 'modernization' approach. For example, policies regulating water use became an important issue in Mexico City—towards the end of the century, new fountains and a public bathhouse were constructed, and decrees promoting improved public hygiene were published (Walsh 2018, 36–7). Nonetheless, in a number of areas of New Spain, such as the highly urbanized Puebla-Tlaxcala region or the Valley of Mexico, smallpox remained endemic until the end of the colonial period and also after independence, with at least eight notable outbreaks registered between 1761 and 1861 (Pereiro-Otero 2008, 112; Thompson 1996, 174). The situation in other parts of the viceroyalty often differed in regard to population density, ethnicity, climate, economic structure or administrative penetration. The province (intendancy) of Oaxaca, according to the census of 1790, had 410,000 inhabitants; 88 percent were classified as 'indigenous.' In 1794, up to 30,000 people in Oaxaca were employed in activities related to the cochineal industry (Baskes 2005, 192). Produced from the *dactylopius coccus* insect, the red dye regularly ranked second after silver when it came to Spanish America's revenue sources and most of it came from indigenous communities in Oaxaca (Gabriel 2022; Tarantola 1999, 44–5). While the region was of little relevance to European settlement, it was definitely integrated into wider economic and social networks because of cochineal or textile production. Native groups possessed most of the lands and regularly used the Spanish legal system to support their claims (Hamnett 1971, 51; Hensel 1999, 219–20; Taylor 1974, 397). Religious *cofradías*, in lieu of communities, sometimes controlled indigenous property, and, even though this phenomenon was less significant in Oaxaca compared to other regions, socio-religious activities of *cofradías* and their importance for shaping local identity likely supported traditions of self-determination and might have played a role in responses to anti-contagion measures in 1796/97 (Chance and Taylor 1985, 11–12; Mendoza García 2002, 751–2; Norget 2008, 150–1).

Soon after Spanish officials reported the outbreak of smallpox in Guatemala in 1795, administrators in Oaxaca implemented prohibitions on the import of textiles and cloth from the affected regions because these products were identified as potential carriers of the disease (Ramírez 2012, 211–2). In the summer of 1796, a viceregal decree declared a state of emergency in Oaxaca, Guadalajara, Puebla, Zacatecas, and other regions—effectively placing areas from the Guatemalan border to the mining centers of Northern Mexico under a specific anti-contagion regime. At the same time, clerics started organizing prayers and processions honoring the Virgin Mary or "plague saints" like Sebastian as part of their ideological support for colonial rule (Few 2018, 171; Ramírez 2018, 98; Widmer 1988, 76). The state encouraged activities by Church representatives; 'modernization' policies in Spanish America did not simply aim at repressing religious influences, but rather at integrating them into 'enlightened colonialism.' That the archbishop of Mexico supported religious activities to end the epidemic and, at the same time, promoted the distribution of an informational pamphlet on the advantages of inoculation (*Método claro, sencillo y fácil para practicar la inoculación elaborado por el Real Tribunal del Protomedicato*), is typical for the cooperation of church and secular administration (Agostoni 2011: 460).

Administrators in Oaxaca acted according to the viceregal orders from Mexico City, implemented quarantine measures, and established a children's infirmary. In Teotitlán del Valle, one of Oaxaca's textile production centers, the local Mixtec-Zapotec population initially accepted the new approach of caring for children outside of families and in a state institution, but this attitude changed, and cooperation with Spanish authorities gave way to verbal aggression and physical violence (Ramírez 2012, 213–7). Official strategies aimed at 'total separación' (Secretaría de Estado 1796b, 7r), but placing children in provisional state-run facilities or the construction of separated graveyards for smallpox victims outside regular Christian cemeteries could definitely be seen as undermining the population's idea of self-determination. Historical research has convincingly shown the gendered aspects of indigenous resistance against these measures and that state actions—deliberately or not—threatened the normative social roles of women (Pastor 1987, 404–7; Thompson 1993, 432). Protests against anti-contagion measures in towns like Teotitlán del Valle showed an ambivalence of identity: indigenous inhabitants wanted to bury deceased children in churchyards, thus integrating themselves into the Catholic Spanish realm. On the other hand, regional traditions dating back to pre-colonial times stressed a specific bond between mothers and their offspring which can help in explaining the resistance against treating children in the new infirmaries (Ramírez 2012, 224–35). From a European perspective, anti-quarantine protests were closely linked to ethnicity, a fact that is hardly surprising if we keep in mind the predominantly indigenous settlement of Oaxaca. However, the general quarantine rules and travel bans did not only affect indigenous communities—traders, many of them Europeans, were hit hard as well, with many of them supporting the protests because of economic and financial reasons.

Under pressure by businesspeople, church officials, and indigenous groups, state administrators, starting in November 1796, implemented a new anti-contagion strategy. Variolation, as had been practiced already in 1779 or during the 1780 Guatemalan epidemic, had a lot of advantages compared to quarantine: it could provide long-term protection, did not disturb production and trade, and allowed families to care for sick relatives. Potential disadvantages were fatal infections in about one to two percent of all variolated persons, scarring or transmissions of syphilis (Franco-Paredes, Lammoglia, and Santos-Preciado 2005, 1285). During the second half of the eighteenth century, a number of Spanish physicians such as Timoteo O'Scanlan had published works on the advantages of inoculation as a 'modern' method of fighting smallpox (1784; Consejo de Castilla 1783/1784). Other publications, like Francisco Gil's *Disertación físico-médica*, accepted inoculation as a potential last measure to stop smallpox, but primarily promoted traditional quarantine strategies (1784). Thus it becomes clear that, in the late eighteenth century, the issue of dealing with medical contingencies was a controversial one, and, while there was widespread belief that the crown should and could protect its Amerindian subjects, there was no unanimous position on how to do this.

After the unrest in Teotitlán and judicial actions related to it, authorities changed their anti-contagion approach quite quickly. Already during November 1796, state administrators started a variolation program among the indigenous population and were able to implement it without further resistance; one of the main factors for the immediate acceptance of variolation might have been the fact that, shortly after its introduction, most community and individual travel restrictions and quarantines as well as trade bans in the Intendancy of Oaxaca were lifted (Ramírez 2012, 230). While state-sponsored inoculation protected many inhabitants of Guatemala—where Captain-General Domás y Valle had quickly implemented this measure—and Oaxaca from contracting smallpox, and some areas in the region did not experience an epidemic mainly because of low population density, the disease finally made its way towards Central Mexico in the spring of 1797 (Cook 1939, 946; Lovell 2021, 25). In some cases, local medical experts and officials argued vehemently in favor of inoculation, citing the example of Oaxaca (where the population had resisted quarantine, but accepted inoculation) as a success story while, in a parallel approach, large religious events were staged, some of them financed by the viceroy and his wife (Cooper 1965, 142; Thompson 1993, 437).

## State Subjects and Othering

If we look at the cases of Guatemala (1780) and Oaxaca (1796/97) in the context of imperial policies towards state subjects and official anti-contagion strategies, we can find a number of similarities as well as differences. Both regions had a high above average number of inhabitants defined as 'indigenous.' They lay further from the colonial core region, authorities acted quickly when it came to dealing with a smallpox outbreak, and countermeasures were generally judged as quite effective by contemporary European observers. However, the situation also differed in some respects: eighteenth-century Oaxaca was an economically flourishing region whose "intimate connection with the business networks radiating out of Mexico City is evident" (Hamnett 1994, 43). Many important roads ran through the province while large parts of Guatemala were seen as impenetrable jungle areas. Native elites in Oaxaca, already in the early seventeenth century, had chosen to migrate to the provincial capital, Antequera, to improve their social and legal possibilities, and, while Mixtecs and Zapotecs retained many of their cultural characteristics, Christianity had become a cornerstone of identity by the late eighteenth century (Megged 1991, 478; Wood 1991, 292–3). In peripheral regions of Guatemala, there had been little to no contact between state administrators or clergymen and indigenous Mayan inhabitants. The role played by women, particularly mothers, features prominently in the case of Oaxaca, but not Guatemala in 1780; however, during a typhus outbreak in 1795, Maya women in Santa María Nebaj in northwestern Guatemala held a number of Spaniards hostage to force the burial of diseased children inside the village church (Dunn 1995, 596–601). Finally, and quite obviously, the approaches to dealing with smallpox in the two cases differed: in Guatemala, inoculation was promoted by the state, church, medical experts, and a number of indigenous leaders. Sixteen years later, authorities in Oaxaca implemented not an inoculation, but a quarantine and isolation program. Only after popular protests did political leaders change their strategy, settling on an inoculation campaign that proved to be effective and acceptable to the indigenous populace.

When it comes to the question of how the colonial state dealt with supporting and/or integrating groups defined by the imperial administration as Other during the course of anti-contagion policies, we can again see an ambivalent picture. In Spain's colonial empire the issue of race, ethnicity, and social hierarchization loomed large—unsurprisingly, Mexico and Guatemala made no exception. However, during the eighteenth century, one of the most striking expressions of an (imagined) racially and socially stratified order was to be found almost exclusively in New Spain: *casta* paintings. These paintings—usually created as commissioned works for members of the Spanish and/or colonial elite—show a deep concern with biopolitics: they are not about individuals, but about stereotypes of race and class; and they only make sense when read against the background of a colonial power ruling over a population deliberately differentiated and othered by state policies.

While Spanish America was officially divided into two distinct ethno-social *repúblicas* (*de los indios* and *de los españoles*), "the mixing of blood produced a tertiary, intermediate people identified as castas" (Carrera 1998, 38). *Casta* paintings usually consist of a series of images depicting a man and a woman with their offspring; possible ethnic combinations that derive from a mixing of Europeans, Africans, and Amerindians are shown to the degree that, for example, even fifth-degree derivations are assigned specific characteristics and names (Jiménez del Val 2009, 2). Although "*casta* paintings were likely not part of coordinated effort at persuasion, they still function as persuasive means of identification in the Burkean sense, leading toward an alignment of interests or senses of self" (Olson 2009, 313). While it is clear that persons—or stereotypes—depicted in these paintings indeed were a part of Spanish colonial society, hierarchization and skepticism towards certain ethnic groups (or 'race mixing' in general) are obvious. Paintings by Miguel Cabrera or Francisco Clapera show physical violence between partners; spatial settings, "bodily and facial features, occupational tools, clothing, animals and fruits are all used to represent degenerate characters" (Guzauskyte 2009, 177–8). In these paintings, however, violence is used either among non-Europeans or by non-Europeans towards Europeans, often describing a world turned upside down because of broken racial barriers: for a colonial empire, the idea of Africans, *castas* or other marginalized groups (literally) attacking a European symbolized an attack on all Europeans and on the social order of the imperial realm.

Ethnicity turns out to be a central topic in social discourses in *Nueva España*, but certainly not the only one. As mentioned earlier, both Oaxaca and Guatemala featured large indigenous populations, but even rural parts of Oaxaca were integrated into the empire, while wide swaths of Guatemala like the Cuchumatán Highlands were basically *terra incognita* for Spaniards. From an administrative point of view, the indigenous inhabitants of Oaxaca could be recognized as Other because of their status as *indio/india* and surviving elements of Mixtec or Zapotec culture; at the same time, however, there was no obvious need to bring them 'into the fold' of colonial society. They already had been integrated via state bureaucracy, Catholicism, trade connections as well as—in the case of the provincial capital—a large proportion of 'Spanish' inhabitants (29.9 percent in 1777), many inter-ethnic marriages, and a relevant *mestizo* and *casta* population (Chance 1975, 219; Rabell 1991, 276; Taylor 1974, 399). In Guatemala, on the other hand, the colonial state, represented in the

21 provinces by only two or three dozen salaried officials, did indeed see the necessity to integrate Mayan populations as well as the possibility to do so through public health policy. José Flores, the doctor leading the inoculation campaign, relied heavily on priests, trusted members of indigenous communities, and the use of indigenous languages to make the strategy work (Few 2010, 530; Patch 1994, 81). In general, a measure like inoculation—or vaccination—can be easily acceptable since it allows people to almost immediately continue their usual way of life; the main impediment to the Guatemalan inoculation program of 1780 was not popular resistance, but the almost nonexistent infrastructure in large parts of the administrative region (Bhattacharya and Brimnes 2009, 10; Few 2010, 528). The areas reached by the anti-smallpox campaign showed the effectiveness of inoculation: in Chiapas, 8,900 persons were inoculated; only 218 died during the epidemic, while 3,100 non-inoculated inhabitants reportedly succumbed to smallpox (Secretaría de Estado 1796c, 1r–2r).

Although some officials in Guatemala, during the next large smallpox outbreak (1794/95), still feared that Mayan 'barbarians' would kill them if their children died after inoculation, physical violence featured much more prominently during the 1796/97 Oaxaca *tumulto* and even led to the deployment of militiamen to curb anti-quarantine protests (Few 2010, 531; Secretaría de Estado 1796a; Secretaría de Estado 1797, 153r). According to Spanish official Esteban Melgar, inhabitants of Teotitlán were unwilling to accept European-style anti-smallpox measures and, influenced by pre-colonial customs, hindered their implementation (Ramírez 2012, 218). Protests, however, were neither directed against the Spanish crown nor based on some kind of 'irrational' behavior: the indigenous population acted according to local traditions of biological relationships as well as socioeconomic needs in the context of an early modern market economy. Disorder was "of the small, spontaneous, highly localised kind frequently found in ancien régime societies" (McFarlane 1995, 313). Punishments were in no way comparable to the ones enforced after New Spain's most notorious unrest, the 1692 Mexico City riots (Exbalin 2016, 227).

Failures in communicating the specific anti-smallpox measures might have played a role in creating an unfavorable reaction in Oaxaca. The colonial state did not necessarily frame the local population as Other at the beginning of the quarantine and isolation measures in 1796—measures taken simply reflected a (quite traditional) European-style approach to public hygiene and dealing with contagion (Ramírez 2012, 212–14); notions about local populations as "the Other [that] cannot be subsumed by sameness" (Jáuregui 2009, 63) are absent. At the same time, officials failed to understand that indigenous communities in Oaxaca differed from many other groups that had effectively been destroyed as cultural and socioeconomic actors. Indigenous landholding and control over the production of a highly valued resource like cochineal, over generations, had fostered self-confidence and self-determination. Only after indigenous communities had reacted in an unexpected and unwanted fashion, officials like Esteban Melgar framed *indios* and *indias* as pre-modern, antagonistic, and irrational Other opposed to the 'enlightened' and humanist policies of the crown (Melgar 1796, 44). This framing, however, did not prove sustainable: a strategy deemed even more 'enlightened'—inoculation of the populace—was quickly accepted throughout communities that, only weeks earlier, had attacked representatives of the colonial state. Quite obviously, protests had not been rooted in animosities towards scientific methods, but in emotional as well as pragmatic reactions focusing on individual safety and the socioeconomic well-being of communities. "Emotions are also tied to moral values, often arising from perceived infractions on moral rules" (Jasper 1998, 401); there is little doubt that taking children from families and putting them into infirmaries was seen as such an infraction, as was the burial of young smallpox victims in a separated graveyard. Criticism of quarantine measures based on economic grounds was not limited to indigenous persons, but also included European manufacturers or merchants, individuals undoubtedly seen as 'rational.' At the same time, clergymen in the region also vehemently opposed forced isolation, especially when it came to children (Ramírez 2012, 218–30). The specific framework of protest made it more necessary, but, at the same time, more acceptable, to the crown, to modify its anti-contagion policy. It seems questionable if protests by indigenous villagers alone would have led to a rapid change in strategy; however, shared interests of European merchants, Catholic clerics, and the indigenous communities not only resulted in intense pressure on the state, but also in the possibility to placate a number of important 'players' at once. While indigenous actors were characterized by some officials as being inimical to the policies and the crown (Melgar 1796: 23), it was quite clear from the beginning that civil unrest did not aim at ending Spanish rule—in fact, the villagers of Teotitlán del Valle had started their protests by hiring a European attorney in the provincial capital (Taylor 1974, 411). It is obvious that indigenous people could easily be framed as ethnic Other, but the ethnic order and hierarchization of the empire did not discourage them from using the Spanish legal system. Thus, the events might also clearly show the limits of a simple dichotomy of colonizer and colonized: colonial subjects classified as 'indigenous' were, *per definitionem*, perceived as being different from Europeans (which, of course, also served the purpose of supporting Spanish rule); at the same time, however, the same courts that would have upheld the ethnic divisions within the empire allowed indigenous groups to resist colonial policies. While Spanish attorneys and Mixtec villagers might have had few things in common, there existed a pragmatic understanding that they were both parts of the same realm, and that Amerindians could hire an attorney without giving up their identity, just like the attorney could defend indigenous interests without jeopardizing his own ethnic *calidad*.

Although anti-smallpox policies in 1780 and 1796 primarily targeted indigenous populations, the settings, strategies, and outcomes differed—and so did the framing of these populations as a non-European Other. On the peripheries of the colonial state in Guatemala, othering Mayan subjects was relatively easy and part of long-standing traditions of cultural contact (or its absence). The inoculation campaign clearly followed a biopolitical top-down approach embedded in a larger strategy of administratively penetrating the region; nonetheless, it seems plausible that effectively communicating these actions among people outside an imperial framework helped facilitate their acceptance. In eighteenth-century Oaxaca, indigenous inhabitants were primarily seen as Other because of their status as *indio* and *india*, not so much because of their lifestyle, settlement patterns or the degree of transcultural contact. Presumed familiarity might have concealed the fact that Mixtecs and Zapotecs in the area were able to act as self-confident non-Europeans. Framing them as Other was, in large parts, a hostile reaction to these populations not accepting the initial anti-smallpox strategies implemented by the colonial administration.

## Works Cited

Agostoni, Claudia. 2011. "Estrategias, actores, promesas y temores en las campañas de vacunación antivariolosa en México: de Porfiriato a la Postrevolución (1880–1940)." *Revista Ciência & Saúde Coletiva* 16, no. 2 (February): 459–70.

Andrieu, Chloé. 2010. "Flexibilité de l'organisation des espaces funéraires dans un village maya du Chiapas aux XVIII<sup>e</sup> et XIX<sup>e</sup> Siècles." *Journal de la Société des Américanistes* 96, no. 2: 253–65.

Baldwin, Peter. 1999. *Contagion and the State in Europe 1830–1930*. Cambridge: Cambridge University Press.

Barquet, Nicolau, and Pere Domingo. 1997. "Smallpox: The Triumph over the Most Terrible of the Ministers of Death." *Annals of Internal Medicine* 127, no. 8 (October): 635–42.

Baskes, Jeremy. 2005. "Colonial Institutions and Cross-Cultural Trade: *Repartimiento* Credit and Indigenous Production of Cochineal in Eighteenth-Century Oaxaca, Mexico." *The Journal of Economic History* 65, no. 1 (March): 186–210.

Bazin, Hervé. 2000. *The Eradication of Smallpox*. Translated by Andrew Morgan and Genise Morgan. New York: Academic Press.

Behbehani, Abbas M. 1983. "The Smallpox Story: Life and Death of an Old Disease." *Microbiological Review* 47, no. 4 (December): 455–509.

Bhattacharya, Sanjoy, and Niels Brimnes. 2009. "Introduction: Simultaneously Global and Local; Reassessing Smallpox Vaccination and Its Spread, 1789–1900." *Bulletin of the History of Medicine* 83, no. 1 (Spring): 1–16.

Brooks, Francis J. 1993. "Revising the Conquest of Mexico: Smallpox, Sources, and Populations." *The Journal of Interdisciplinary History* 24, no. 1 (Summer): 1–29.

Carmichael, Ann G., and Arthur M. Silverstein. 1987. "Smallpox in Europe before the Seventeenth Century: Virulent Killer or Benign Disease?" *Journal of the History of Medicine and Allied Sciences* 42, no. 2 (April): 147–68.

Carrera, Magali M. 1998. "Locating Race in Late Colonial Mexico." *Art Journal* 57, no. 3 (Autumn): 36–45.

Chance, John K. 1975. "The Colonial Latin American City: Preindustrial or Capitalist?" *Urban Anthropology* 4, no. 3 (Fall): 211–28.

Chance, John K., and William B. Taylor. 1985. "Cofradías and Cargos: An Historical Perspective on the Mesoamerican Civil-Religious Hierarchy." *American Ethnologist* 12, no. 1: 1–26.

Chuchiak, John F. IV. 2005. "In Servitio Dei: Fray Diego de Landa, the Franciscan Order, and the Return of the Extirpation of Idolatry in the Colonial Diocese of Yucatán, 1573–1579." *The Americas* 61, no. 4 (April): 611–46.

Clendinnen, Inga. 1982. "Disciplining the Indians: Franciscan Ideology and Missionary Violence in Sixteenth-Century Yucatán." *Past & Present* 94 (February): 27–48.

Consejo de Castilla. 1783/1784. *Licencia de impresión de 'Prática moderna de la inoculación: Con varias observaciones y reflexiones...' solicitada por su autor Timoteo*

*O-Scanlan*. ES.28079.AHN/Consejos, 5547, 41. Archivo Histórico Nacional, Madrid, Spain.

Cook, Noble David. 2002. "Sickness, Starvation, and Death in Early Hispaniola." *The Journal of Interdisciplinary History* 32, no. 3 (Winter): 349–86.

Cook, S. F. 1939. "The Smallpox Epidemic of 1797 in Mexico." *Bulletin of the History of Medicine* 7, no. 8 (October): 937–69.

Cooper, Donald B. 1965. *Epidemic Disease in Mexico City 1761–1813: An Administrative, Social, and Medical Study*. Austin: University of Texas Press.

Crocker, Rebecca. 2014. "Healing on the Edge: The Construction of Medicine on the Jesuit Frontier of Northern New Spain." *Journal of the Southwest* 56, no. 2 (Summer): 293–318.

Curtin, Philip D. 1993. "Disease Exchange across the Tropical Atlantic." *History and Philosophy of the Life Sciences* 15, no. 3: 329–56.

De Bevoise, Ken. 1990. "Until God Knows When: Smallpox in the Late-Colonial Philippines." *Pacific Historical Review* 59, no. 2 (May): 149–85.

De Burgos, Hugo. 2014. "Contemporary Transformations of Indigenous Medicine and Ethnic Identity." *Anthropologica* 56, no. 2: 399–413.

Díaz-Polanco, Héctor, and Araceli Burguete. 1989. "Sociedad colonial y rebelión indígena en el istmo de Tehuantepec." *Boletín de Antropología Americana* 20 (December): 99–124.

Dunn, Alvis E. 1995. "A Cry at Daybreak: Death, Disease, and Defense of Community in a Highland Ixil-Mayan Village." *Ethnohistory* 42, no. 4 (Autumn): 595–606.

Eliade, Mircea. 1951. *Le chamanisme et les techniques archaïques de l'exstase*. Paris: Payot.

Exbalin, Arnaud. 2016. "Riot in Mexico City: A Challenge to the Colonial Order?" *Urban History* 43, no. 2 (May): 215–31.

Few, Martha. 2010. "Circulating Smallpox Knowledge: Guatemalan Doctors, Maya Indians and Designing Spain's Smallpox Vaccination Expedition, 1780–1803." *The British Journal for the History of Science* 43, no. 4 (December): 519–37.

———. 2012. "Medical Humanitarianism and Smallpox Inoculation in Eighteenth-Century Guatemala." *Historical Social Research/Historische Sozialforschung* 37, no. 3: 303–17.

———. 2018. "'Speaking with the Fire': The Inquisition Confronts Mesoamerican Divination to Treat Child Illness in Sixteenth-Century Guatemala." *Early Science and Medicine* 23, no. 1/2: 159–76.

Foster, George M. 1987. "On the Origin of Humoral Medicine in Latin America." *Medical Anthropology Quarterly N. S.* 1, no. 4 (December): 355–93.

Franco-Paredes, Carlos, Lorena Lammoglia, and José Ignacio Santos-Preciado. 2005. "The Spanish Royal Philanthropic Expedition to Bring Smallpox Vaccination to the New World and Asia in the 19th Century." *Clinical Infectious Diseases* 41, no. 9 (November): 1285–89.

Fredrick, Sharonah. 2021. "Mayan and Andean Medicine and Urban Space in the Spanish Americas." *Renaissance and Reformation / Renaissance et Réforme* 44, no. 2 (Spring): 147–81.

Frühsorge, Lars. 2011. "Getanzte Erinnerung und der Traum von einem indianischen Königtum: Spuren einer kolonialzeitlichen Heilserwartungsbewegung im Hochland Guatemalas." *Anthropos* 106, no. 1: 87–97.

Gabriel, Martin. 2019. "Staatsräson und Militärreform. Alejandro O'Reilly, Spanisch-Amerika und die Modernisierung eines Weltreiches (1763–1770)." *Pallasch: Zeitschrift für Militärgeschichte* 67: 23–34.

———. 2022. "Eine Laus erobert die Welt. Die Koschenilleschildlaus (Dactylopius coccus) und das 'rote Gold' Neuspaniens." *Amerindian Research* 17, no. 4: 212–23.

Gil, Francisco. 1784. *Disertacion fisico-médica, en la qual se prescribe un método seguro para preservar a los pueblos de viruelas hasta lograr la completa extincion de ellas en todo el reyno.* Madrid: Joaquín Ibarra.

Guzauskyte, Evelina. 2009. "Fragmented Borders, Fallen Men, Bestial Women: Violence in the Casta Paintings of Eighteenth-Century New Spain." *Bulletin of Spanish Studies* 86, no. 2 (March): 175–204.

Hämäläinen, Pekka. 2010. "The Politics of Grass: European Expansion, Ecological Change, and Indigenous Power in the Southwest Borderlands." *The William and Mary Quarterly* 67, no. 2 (April): 173–208.

Hamnett, Brian R. 1971. "Dye Production, Food Supply, and the Laboring Population of Oaxaca, 1750–1820." *The Hispanic American Historical Review* 51, no. 1 (February): 51–78.

———. 1994. "Between Bourbon Reforms and Liberal Reforma: The Political Economy of a Mexican Province; Oaxaca, 1750–1850." In *The Political Economy of Spanish America in the Age of Revolution, 1750–1850*, edited by Kenneth Andrien and Lyman L. Johnson, 39–62. Albuquerque: University of New Mexico Press.

Hensel, Silke. 1999. "Los orígines del federalismo en México: Una perspectiva desde la provincia de Oaxaca de finales del siglo XVIII a la Primera República." *Ibero-amerikanisches Archiv* 25, no. 3/4: 215–37.

Hernández Sáenz, Luz María. 2000. "Medicos criollos y cirujanos peninsula-res: Criollo Nationalism and the Medical Profession in Colonial Mexico." *Canadian Journal of Latin American and Caribbean Studies / Revue canadienne des études latino-américaines et caraïbes* 25, no. 49: 33–51.

Hill, Robert M. 1989. "Social Organization by Decree in Colonial Highland Guatemala." *Ethnohistory* 36, no. 2 (Spring): 170–98.

Hinojosa, Servando Z. 2002. "'The Hands Know': Bodily Engagement and Med-ical Impasse in Highland Maya Bonesetting." *Medical Anthropology Quarterly* 16, no. 1 (March): 22–40.

Janssens, Uta. 1981. "Matthieu Maty and the Adoption of Inoculation for Small-pox in Holland." *Bulletin of the History of Medicine* 55, no. 2 (Summer): 246–56.

Jasper, James M. 1998. "The Emotions of Protest: Affective and Reactive Emo-tions in and around Social Movements." *Sociological Forum* 13, no. 3 (Septem-ber): 397–424.

Jáuregui, Carlos A. 2009. "Cannibalism, the Eucharist, and Criollo Subjects." In *Creole Subjects in the Americas: Empires, Texts, Identities*, edited by Ralph Bauer and José Antonio Mazzotti, 61–100. Chapel Hill: University of North Car-olina Press.

Jáuregui, Carlos A., and David Solodkow. 2018. "Biopolitics and the Farming (of) Life in Bartolomé de las Casas." In *Bartolomé de las Casas, O.P.: History, Philosophy and Theology in the Age of European Expansion*, edited by David T. Orique and Rady Roldán-Figueroa, 127–66. London: Brill.

Jiménez del Val, Nasheli. 2009. "Pinturas de Casta: Mexican Caste Paintings, a Foucauldian Reading." *New Readings* 10 (January): 1–17. http://doi.org/10.1 8573/newreadings.67.

Jones, David S. 2003. "Virgin Soils Revisited." *The William and Mary Quarterly* 60, no. 4 (October): 703–42.

Jones, Eric E. 2014. "Spatiotemporal Analysis of Old World Diseases in North America, A.D. 1519–1807." *American Antiquity* 79, no. 3 (July): 487–506.

Kastoryano, Riva. 2010. "Codes of Otherness." *Social Research* 77, no. 1 (Spring): 79–100.

Kaya, İrfan. 2018. "A Postcolonial Reading on Eurocentrism, Otherization and Orientalist Discourse in Sociological Thought and its Criticism." *ULUM Journal of Religious Inquiries* 1, no. 1 (July): 163–88.

Livi-Bacci, Massimo. 2006. "The Depopulation of America after the Conquest." *Population and Development Review* 32, no. 2 (June): 199–232.

López de Mariscal, Blanca. 2008. "El drama demográfico de la Nueva España en el siglo XVI: El espacio de la mujer." In *Persistencia y cambio: Acercamientos a la historia de las mujeres en México*, edited by Lucia Melgar, 79–97. Mexico City: El Colegio de Mexico.

Lovell, W. George. 1988. "Surviving Conquest: The Maya of Guatemala in Historical Perspective." *Latin American Research Review* 23, no. 2: 25–57.

———. 1992. "'Heavy Shadows and Black Night': Disease and Depopulation in Colonial Spanish America." *Annals of the Association of American Geographers* 82, no. 3 (September): 426–43.

———. 2021. "'Destroying Generation after Generation': Outbreaks of Smallpox in the Cuchumatán Highlands of Guatemala (1780–1810)." *Storicamente* 17, no. 3: 1–33.

Mark, Catherine, and José G. Rigau-Pérez. 2009. "The World's First Immunization Campaign: The Spanish Smallpox Vaccine Expedition, 1803–1813." *Bulletin of the History of Medicine* 83, no. 1 (Spring): 63–94.

Mayer, Karl Herbert. 2015. "A Maya curandera in Seibal, Petén, Guatemala." *Mexicon* 37, no. 5 (October): 105–8.

McCaa, Robert. 1995. "Spanish and Nahuatl Views on Smallpox and Demographic Catastrophe in Mexico." *The Journal of Interdisciplinary History* 25, no. 3 (Winter): 397–431.

McFarlane, Anthony. 1995. "Rebellions in Late Colonial Spanish America: A Comparative Perspective." *Bulletin of Latin American Research* 14, no. 3 (September): 313–38.

McNeill, J. R. 1999. "Ecology, Epidemics and Empires: Environmental Change and the Geopolitics of Tropical America, 1600–1825." *Environment and History* 5, no. 2 (June): 175–84.

Megged, Amos. 1991. "Accommodation and Resistance of Elites in Transition: The Case of Chiapa in Early Colonial Mesoamerica." *The Hispanic American Historical Review* 71, no. 3 (August): 477–500.

———. 1992. "The Rise of Creole Identity in Early Colonial Guatemala: Differential Patterns in Town and Countryside." *Social History* 17, no. 3 (October): 421–40.

Melgar, Esteban. 1796. *Letter to Antonio de Mora y Peysal*. Epidemias 15, 2. Archivo General de la Nación, Mexico City, Mexico.

Mendoza García, Edgar. 2002. "El ganado comunal en la Mixteca Alta: De la época colonial al siglo XX: El caso de Tepelmeme." *Historia Mexicana* 51, no. 4 (April–June): 749–85.

Miño Grijalva, Manuel. 2012. "El Otoño de la muerte: La crisis demográfica de 1779 en la Ciudad de México." *Historia Mexicana* 62, no. 2 (October–December): 591–626.

Montero Lazcano, Mara Yolanda. 2020. "Indigenismos en el discurso médico de Guatemala del siglo XVIII: El caso de la Instrucción sobre el modo de practicar la inoculación de las viruelas de José Felipe Flores." *Études romanes de Brno* 41, no. 2: 41–51.

Moreno Okuno, Alejandro T., and Daniel Ventosa-Santaulària. 2010. "Fall in the Indian Population after the Arrival of the Spaniards: Diseases or Exploitation?" *Investigación Económica* 69 (April–June): 87–104.

Motolinía [Fray Toribio de Benavente]. 1971. *Memoriales o libro de las cosas de la Nueva España y de las naturales de ella*. Edited by Edmundo O'Gorman. Mexico City: Universidad Nacional Autónoma de México.

Moynihan, Donald, and Gregory Porumbescu. 2020. "Trump's 'Chinese virus' Slur Makes People Blame Chinese Americans. But Others Blame Trump." *Washington Post*. September 16, 2020. https://www.washingtonpost.com/politics/2020/09/16/trumps-chinese-virus-slur-makes-some-people-bla me-chinese-americans-others-blame-trump/.

Muñoz Camargo, Diego. 1966. *Historia de Tlaxcala*. 2nd ed. Edited by Alfredo Chavero. Guadalajara: Aviña Levy.

Newman, Marshall T. 1976. "Aboriginal New World Epidemiology and Medical Care, and the Impact of Old World Disease Imports." *Journal of Physical Anthropology* 45, no. 3 (November): 667–72.

Newson, Linda A. 2006. "Medical Practice in Early Colonial Spanish America: A Prospectus." *Bulletin of Latin American Research* 25, no. 3 (July): 367–91.

Norget, Kristin. 2008. "Hard Habits to Baroque: Catholic Church and Popular-Indigenous Religious Dialogue in Oaxaca, Mexico." *Revista Canadiense de Estudios Hispánicos* 33, no. 1: 131–58.

Olson, Christa. 2009. "Casta Painting and the Rhetorical Body." *Rhetoric Society Quarterly* 39, no. 4 (Fall): 307–30.

Orellana, Sandra L. 1981. "Idols and Idolatry in Highland Guatemala." *Ethnohistory* 28, no. 2 (Spring): 157–77.

O'Scanlan, Timoteo. 1784. *Practica moderna de la inoculación: Con varias observaciones y reflexiones fundadas en ella, precedidas de un discurso sobre la utilidad de esta operacion y un compendio historico de su origen y de su estado actual, particularmente en España: Con un catalogo de algunos inoculados*. Madrid: Miguel Copin.

Palma Murga, Gustavo. 2007. "Between Fidelity and Pragmatism: Guatemala's Commercial Elite Responds to Bourbon Reforms on Trade and Contraband." In *Politics, Economy, and Society in Bourbon Central America, 1759–1821*, edited by Jordana Dym and Christophe Belaubre, 101–27. Boulder: University Press of Colorado.

Pastor, Rodolfo. 1987. *Campesinos y reformas: La mixteca, 1700–1856.* Mexico City: El Colegio de México.

Patch, Robert W. 1994. "Imperial Politics and Local Economy in Colonial Central America 1670–1770." *Past & Present* 143 (May): 77–107.

———. 1996. "Sacraments and Disease in Mérida, Yucatán, Mexico, 1648–1727." *The Historian* 58, no. 4 (Summer): 731–43.

Pereiro-Otero, José Manuel. 2008. "Conquistas vi(r)olentas y vacunas independentistas: Andrés Bello y Manuel José Quintana ante la enfermedad de la colonia." *Hispanic Review* 76, no. 2 (Spring): 109–33.

Pitarch, Pedro. 2007. "The Political Uses of Maya Medicine: Civil Organizations in Chiapas and the Ventriloquism Effect." *Social Analysis* 51, no. 2 (Summer): 185–206.

Pugh, Timothy W. 2009. "Contagion and Alterity: Kowoj Maya Appropriations of European Objects." *American Anthropologist N. S.* 111, no. 3 (September): 373–86.

Rabell, Cecilia Andrea. 1991. "Estructuras de la población y características de los jefes de los grupos domésticos en la ciudad de Antequera (Oaxaca), 1777." In *Familias novohispanas, siglos XVI al XIX*, edited by Pilar Gonzalbo Aizpuru, 273–98. Mexico City: El Colegio de México.

Ramenofsky, Ann F., Alicia K. Wilbur, and Anne C. Stone. 2003. "Native American Disease History: Past, Present and Future Directions." *World Archaeology* 35, no. 2 (October): 241–57.

Ramírez, Paul. 2012. "'Like Herod's Massacre': Quarantines, Bourbon Reform, and Popular Protest in Oaxaca's Smallpox Epidemic, 1796–1797." *The Americas* 69, no. 2 (October): 203–35.

———. 2018. *Enlightened Immunity: Mexico's Experiments with Disease Prevention in the Age of Reason.* Stanford: Stanford University Press.

Rigau-Pérez, José G. 1982. "Smallpox Epidemics in Puerto Rico during the Pre-vaccine Era (1518–1803)." *Journal of the History of Medicine and Allied Sciences* 37, no. 4 (October): 423–38.

Riley, James C. 2010. "Smallpox and American Indians Revisited." *Journal of the History of Medicine and Allied Sciences* 65, no. 4 (October): 445–77.

Sampeck, Kathryn E. 2014. "From Ancient Altepetl to Modern Municipios: Surveying as Power in Colonial Guatemala." *International Journal of Historical Archaeology* 18, no. 1 (March): 175–203.

Sandberg, Eric T., Mark W. Kline, and William T. Shearer. 1996. "The Secondary Immunodeficiences." In *Immunologic Disorders in Infants & Children*, 4th ed., edited by E. Richard Stiehm, 553–601. Philadelphia: Saunders.

Secretaría de Estado y del Despacho de Estado. 1796a. *Carta to Manuel Godoy, Príncipe de la Paz*. ES.41091.AGI/22/Estado, 25, 54. Archivo General de Indias. Sevilla, Spain.

Secretaría de Estado y del Despacho de Estado. 1796b. *Epidemias de viruelas en Teutitlán*. ES.47161.AGS/SGU/LEG, 6974, 16. Archivo General de Simancas. Simancas, Spain.

Secretaría de Estado y del Despacho de Estado. 1796c. *Letter to Manuel Godoy, Príncipe de la Paz*. ES.41091.AGI/22/Estado, 37, 55. Archivo General de Indias. Sevilla, Spain.

Secretaría de Estado y del Despacho de Guerra. 1797. *Letter to the Viceroy of New Spain*. ES.47161.AGS/ SGU, LEG, 6974, 16, Archivo General de Simancas. Simancas, Spain.

Sesia, Paola M. 1996. "'Women Come Here on Their Own When They Need to.' Prenatal Care, Authoritative Knowledge, and Maternal Health in Oaxaca." *Medical Anthropology Quarterly* 10, no. 2 (June): 121–40.

Smith, Michael M. 1974. "The 'Real Expedición Marítima de la Vacuna' in New Spain and Guatemala." *Transactions of the American Philosophical Society* 64, no. 1: 1–74.

Tarantola, Giulia. 1999. "Cochenille et Indigo en Méso-Amérique (1770–1870)." *Études rurales* 151, no. 2 (July–December): 43–9.

Taylor, William B. 1974. "Landed Society in New Spain: A View from the South." *The Hispanic American Historical Review* 54, no. 3 (August): 387–413.

Tedlock, Dennis. 1993. "Torture in the Archives: Mayans meet Europeans." *American Anthropologist* 95, no. 1 (March): 139–52.

Thompson, Angela. 2018. "Smallpox: Ensuring the Destruction of Armies in Colonial New Spain and Peru, 1518–1625." In *Epidemics and War: The Impact of Disease on Major Conflicts in History*, edited by Rebecca M. Seaman, 129–46. Santa Barbara: ABC-Clio.

Thompson, Angela T. 1993. "To Save the Children: Smallpox Inoculation, Vaccination, and Public Health in Guanajuato, Mexico, 1797–1840." *The Americas* 49, no. 4 (April): 431–55.

——— . 1996. "Mexico's Other Wars: Epidemics, Disease, and Public Health in Guanajuato, 1810–1867." *Annales de démographie historique*: 169–94.

Veblen, Thomas T. 1977. "Native Population Decline in Totonicapán, Guatemala." *Annals of the Association of American Geographers* 67, no. 4 (December): 484–99.

Viqueira, Juan Pedro. 1994. "Tributo y sanidad en Chiapas (1680–1721)." *Historia Mexicana* 44, no. 2 (October): 237–67.

Waldstein, Anna, and Cameron Adams. 2006. "The Interface between Medical Anthropology and Medical Ethnobiology." *The Journal of the Royal Anthropological Institute* 12: 95–118.

Walsh, Casey. 2018. *Virtuous Waters: Mineral Springs, Bathing, and Infrastructure in Mexico*. Oakland: University of California Press.

Widmer, Rolf. 1988. "Política sanitaria y lucha social en Tehuantepec, 1795–1796." *Historias* 21, no. 2 (October): 71–90.

Wood, Stephanie. 1991. "Adopted Saints: Christian Images in Nahua Testaments of Late Colonial Toluca." *The Americas* 47, no. 3 (January): 259–93.

# 4. 'Civilizing the Natives' with Modern Medicine: Strategies of Othering in the Implementation of Public Hygiene in Japan-Ruled Taiwan (1895-1945)

*Anke Scherer*

Reports about the handling of the COVID-19 pandemic in Japan often mention the widespread awareness of hygiene and its importance in daily life.[1] Practices such as wearing masks to prevent the spread of germs as well as an omnipresent emphasis on cleanliness are culturally learned and socially reinforced virtues in modern Japan. In contrast to cultural essentialist approaches that connect these practices to indigenous traditions based on religious concepts of purity (Scherer 2019), the history of the development of a modern concept of hygiene in Japan shows that these practices are the result of a process of internalization and application of medical knowledge that is an integral part of the country's modernization process in the second half of the nineteenth century (Joshi and Tewari 2003). This process, however, was dominated by Japan's endeavor to be not only recognized as a civilized nation by Western countries, but also to be taken seriously as a player on the stage of global imperialism in the nineteenth and twentieth century. The construction of today's super-modern country, well prepared to fight a medical challenge like the COVID-19 pandemic,[2] owes a lot to the importance that was given to the eradication of diseases, and the improvement of hygiene, sanitation,

---

[1]    Compare for example a study about COVID-19 responses in South Korea and Japan in which the authors conclude that "[d]espite the rather loose and cautious policy coordination, it should also be noted that citizens' self-restraint and their adherence to social norms and strong awareness of public hygiene are key factors contributing to the effectiveness of the Japanese government's policies" (Moon et al. 2021, 665).

[2]    The 2021 Global Health Security (GHS) Index which measures the capacities of 195 countries to prepare for epidemics and pandemics has ranked Japan as number 18.

and medical education as a parameter for civilization in the formative years of modern Japan. This national identity was formed in a process in which the modernizing country compared itself in an imperialistic context with neighboring countries, resulting in its self-perception as the leading civilization in East Asia and in turn triggered a colonial expansion (Myers and Peattie 1984).

The construction of a modern Japanese nation comprised a clear definition of the country's territory. In this process, the northern island of Hokkaidō, formerly loosely attached to one of the domains of feudal Japan but inhabited by non-Japanese, was fully colonized in the second half of the nineteenth century and made into one of the four main Japanese islands (Boyle 2016). In 1895, the island of Taiwan became Japan's first overseas colony. Although the acquisition of the island was not the intended outcome of the Sino-Japanese War (1894–1895), which had been fought over influence on the Korean peninsula, the relatively inexperienced colonizer Japan nevertheless attempted to turn the newly acquired territory into a showcase of colonial management to prove Japan's rightful membership in the group of Western 'civilized nations' (Hée 2014). "Japanese Attitudes Towards Colonialism" have already been extensively scrutinized by Mark Peattie in his article with the same title (1984). His analysis discusses the paternalistic approach to the people colonized by the Japanese, who claimed to introduce them to the benefits of 'civilization and enlightenment' (*bunmei kaika*, the Japanese slogan for modernization after 1868) but leaves out the colonial practice that resulted from these attitudes. One of the benefits of this modern civilization was the improvement of sanitation and healthcare. The fact that "investment in public health and education made the population healthier and better educated" is usually acknowledged as a thoroughly positive outcome of Japanese colonial management of the island (Morgan and Liu 2007, 990). Michael Shiyung Liu's history of medical practices and policies in Japan-ruled Taiwan covers the many aspects of the establishment of a modern medical system and convincingly shows that "[i]ntroducing scientific medicine and a public health system to Taiwan was a way in which Japan could claim its modernity and build a colony as its Western counterparts had done." (2009, 142). David Arnold analyzed this mechanism for British rule in India where the colonial state's response to epidemic disease had far-reaching implications for public health policy and practice. Although he warns that "[t]he colonizing force of Western medicine has to be understood as more than a crude device of imperial self-legitimization" (1993, 292), he contends that "Western medical discourse [...] seemed in many ways to add a new luster and a more authoritative dimension to colonial rule" (293).

As the seemingly benign project to protect or at least cure the Taiwanese population from diseases was closely connected to the justification of Japan's right to colonize the island, this article argues that the colonizers' fight against pandemics employed various strategies of 'othering' the indigenous society in order to emphasize the contrast between the civilized Japanese rulers and the newly colonized islanders to be eventually 'civilized' into hygienic modernity. To show how the framing of the Taiwanese population as dependent upon superior Japanese skills in fighting epidemics worked, the article starts with a short outline of Japan's rapid hygienic modernization after the 1870s and the ensuing emancipation from formerly used methods of disease control and prevention informed by traditional Chinese medicine. The following analysis of 'othering strategies' employed in the process of 'civilizing the natives' with modern medicine scrutinizes practices of the Japanese colonial government of dealing with the sanitary challenges in Taiwan especially in the campaign to eradicate the plague in the 1910s. The success of disease control and improvement of healthcare was regularly recorded in studies and reports about the public hygiene situation in Taiwan, the last of which was published in 1939 (*TSKE* 1939). As it is a summary of the colonizers' forty-year endeavor to introduce the colonized population to scientific standards of modern public hygiene, the topics in the compilation and especially its wording is examined as a documentation of the mindset underlying the othering of the Taiwanese. The analysis sheds light on the execution of what Foucault called biopower in a colonial context and contributes to the understanding of the mechanism of othering in disease control and prevention.

## The 'Hygienic Turn' and Its Impact on Japanese Colonialism

The development of public hygiene concepts was an important element of the modernization in Japan that followed the regime change after the so-called Meiji-Restauration in 1868. This regime change was the result of a prolonged internal crisis and was eventually triggered by the forced opening of the formerly relatively isolated country through US-American pressure in the 1850s. The end of the premodern rule of the Tokugawa shogunate (1600–1867) was followed by a fast westernization and modernization of the political system, the economy and society. However, the opening of several ports to foreign merchants in the 1850s and the ensuing increase of contacts with the outside world also exposed the Japanese population to outbreaks of epidemics, predominately waterborne diseases like cholera, shigellosis, and typhoid (Jannetta 2007; Jannetta 2009). The most devastating disease in this context was cholera, with a massive outbreak in 1858 that was directly connected to the opening of the country (Gramlich-Oka 2009; Yamamoto 1982). Whereas in the last years of Tokugawa rule, cholera, like other diseases, was often believed to be the result of unhappy deities who should be appeased through prayer, amulets, and the like (Johnston 2019, 13), the new Meiji government responded to outbreaks of epidemics with the creation of institutions, laws, and educational campaigns. All of this was based on a new concept of public hygiene, promoted by a leadership that comprised a relatively high number of politicians educated in modern science, especially medicine (Fukuda 1994, 385–93). What they achieved in the late nineteenth century is sometimes called the "hygienic turn" in Japanese history. It did not only improve the livelihood of the domestic population but quickly also became part of the endeavor to raise Japan's status in the international order through the promotion of the image of a civilized country that was at the forefront of medical research and scientific progress to combat the spread of epidemic diseases (Rogaski 2014, 14).

After the acquisition of the island of Taiwan as Japan's first colony in 1895, the island was supposedly turned into a showcase of the civilizing influence of a Japanese colonial administration (Hée 2014). Shinpei Gotō (1857–1929), a politician who was a medical doctor by training and who had studied abroad in Berlin with Robert Koch (1843–1910) and in Munich with Max von Pettenkofer (1818–1901), was the civil governor of the colony from 1898 to 1906 in the decisive phase of the Japanese takeover. He established an approach to colonial administration that emphasized the importance of public hygiene (Kitaoka 2021). Since endemic diseases like malaria, as well as outbreaks of cholera and the plague were among the biggest challenges for the newly arrived colonizers on the tropical island of Taiwan, disease prevention and the establishment of medical facilities to treat the high number of infected Japanese invaders was given high priority in the creation of colonial institutions. This eventually led to the copying of the system of public hygiene that had just been established in Japan (Liu 2011, 169–70). The overall improvement of sanitation, hygiene, and medical standards became one of the main themes with which the Japanese administration used to justify colonialism vis-á-vis the indigenous society. Liu has already shown how the scientific approach to public health was seen as proof of Japan's ability to properly rule a colony vis-á-vis the other colonial powers (2009, 15, 129). What is left out in Liu's argument is the complex construction of Japan's colonial project in Taiwan, where the Japanese were interacting with a Han-Chinese population that had only recently colonized the island themselves and driven the aboriginal tribes to live beyond a rigidly demarcated "savage boundary" in the eastern highlands (Hirano, Veracini, and Roy 2018). Thus, this article builds on Liu's research about the development of Japan's colonial infrastructure but adds the analysis of the ideological mechanisms used to usurp the top position in the colonial hierarchy in Taiwan from the Han-Chinese.

## The Redefinition of Chinese Cultural Heritage

In comparison to other colonial powers, the Japanese in Taiwan encountered a unique ideological problem. Western colonizers acted in a setting where they perceived themselves in a clear hierarchy of civilizations that allowed them to look down on a supposedly primitive indigenous population. In his book *Orientalism*, Edward Said argues that Western attitudes towards the East, particularly the Middle East, have been shaped by a pervasive cultural bias and a long history of colonial domination. Said suggests that the West has constructed an image of the East that is exotic, mysterious, and inferior, using this image to justify imperialist policies and the subjugation of Eastern peoples (1978). This worldview can lead to the othering of colonial subjects in order to justify the power relations between colonizer and the colonized peoples. However, it usually works only without substantial interaction prior to colonization, because then the hegemonic processes of marking the supposed differences between the superior 'We' (the colonizers) and the inferior 'Other' (the indigenous peoples) can neatly follow the logic of a civilizing mission through colonization. The Japanese colonization of the island of Taiwan, however, cannot be easily explained within the framework of Orientalism, not only because both countries geographically belong to the East, but also because both cultures have a long common history (Nomura 1999, 1–2). Historically, China was the regional hegemon in East Asia and exported its culture to its neighbors, among them the Japanese islands. The change in Japanese attitude from a recipient of Chinese cultural features in premodern times to the self-perceived leading civilization in East Asia in the modernization process of the nineteenth and twentieth century required a redefinition of the regional hierarchy of cultures. Thus, the newly acquired Japanese competence in Western, i.e., modern, disease prevention and medicine quickly became the most important "tool of empire" (Arnold 1993) that was first applied in Taiwan and subsequently employed in Japan's further colonial expansion in Asia.

The distancing from the traditional cultural paragon China and the eventual redefinition of Chinese medical knowledge and practice as backward was a process that stretched over several decades. When Japan started its hygienic modernization in the early 1870s, the very word coined to represent the modern concept of public hygiene was taken from a Chinese classic to lend the concept historical depth and credibility.[3] Traditional Chinese medicine was an integral part of medical knowledge and practice in premodern Japan, medical practitioners in seventeenth and eighteenth century Japan saw it as their task to adapt the universal principles of Chinese medicine to the specific Japanese situation (Trambaiolo 2013, 304). In the regional and international development in the late nineteenth and early twentieth century, however, Japan turned from a peripheral country that was proud to have adopted and perfected many traits of Chinese culture into the power that claimed regional hegemony also over China due to its capability to quickly westernize and modernize its political system, its economy, society and, last but not least, its military in contrast to a stagnating China that was an easy prey for outside powers (Beasley 1991).

The island of Taiwan was not exactly the center of Chinese civilization, but rather a long neglected tropical island where Han-Chinese, who had only arrived between a few hundred years and several decades ago, lived in the western lowland with an aboriginal non-Chinese population dwelling in jungles and mountains in the east (Rubinstein 2007). The actual Japanese takeover of the island was followed by more than fifty local uprisings of the local Chinese population, sometimes supported by non-Chinese mountain dwellers (Hée 2012, 51–121). The Japanese landing on the island was first and foremost a military operation, but more dangerous than the attacks by the low-tech guerrilla forces for the professional Japanese soldiers with their modern equipment were the tropical diseases that killed more soldiers than the local resistance (Katz 1996, 209).

---

3    Japanese script is based on Chinese characters whose pronunciation is adapted. The modern Japanese term *eisei* for 'hygiene' meaning 'community health policed with state authority' was adopted from a passage in the Chinese classic *Zhuang Zi* (compiled between the fifth and third century B.C.E.) where this two-character compound pronounced *weisheng* in Chinese means 'guarding life.' See Ozaki (2016, 66) for the discussion about the creation of the neologism *eisei* in Japan.

In a situation where at least the local Chinese population and especially its elite could not easily be framed in the conventional 'othering category' of the 'illiterate uncivilized' often used in colonial contexts, the specific constellation in colonial Taiwan produced as a different strategy the invocation of the scientific concept of public hygiene. In this framework the Japanese colonial government of Taiwan was the agent bringing hygienic modernity to the 'islanders' that lived in the premodern world of traditional Chinese medicine where causes for diseases were often misunderstood and attempts to cure them lacked any modern scientific basis. The transition from a premodern understanding and handling of disease in Japan had only happened in the middle of the nineteenth century during the first phase of the country's modernization process. Whereas early Japanese proponents of the cowpox vaccine in 1850s were met with the staunch opposition of the mainstream of Japanese doctors, who were all trained in Chinese medicine and explained the symptoms of smallpox as the eruption of an innate poison present in patients' bodies at the time of birth and treated them with either "cooling" or "warming" therapy as recommended in ancient Chinese medical tractates (Trambaiolo 2014), from the 1870s onwards the medical profession in Japan was at the forefront of adapting Western scientific standards and reached international recognition in the early twentieth century (Bartholomew 1993, 109). In contrast, Taiwanese medical practitioners remained within the belief system of traditional Chinese medicine. The Taiwanese people, rather than trusting modern medicine, trusted traditional healers and suspected sinister motives behind inoculation programs of the colonial administration. For example, they believed that the administration was attempting to reduce reproduction rates in order to lower the Taiwanese population rate. However, traditional medical practices were unable to help against the widespread parasites, nor were they able to prevent the spread of tropical diseases among the indigenous inhabitants of the new Japanese colony Taiwan. Instead, regular epidemics allowed the colonial administrators, with their modern means and knowledge, to fight these medical problems and justify their rule of the island by turning it into a model colony and showcase of so-called scientific colonialism.

## Institutionalizing Hygiene in Taiwan

In the domestic development of a modern concept of hygiene in Japan, the focus was largely on the university-based German system with scientific training and laboratory work. Bacteriology and germ theory were quickly adopted in Japanese academia. Gotō Shinpei's conviction that disease prevention was closely connected to public and social hygiene anchored the idea in the colonial administration that not only the tropical environment could be a health threat, but that the behavior of the indigenous people was hazardous to their health. Gotō—a self-proclaimed fan of German *Staatsmedizin* (state medicine)—thus created a sanitary police modeled on the German example that was in charge of supervising the compliance with quarantine regulations, sanitary measures, and other provisions for the maintenance of social hygiene in the general public (Liu 2009, 56–84). Consequently, it was the Police Affairs Department of the Governor-General of Taiwan (*Taiwan sōtokufu keimukyoku*) that published, as one of its many reports about this topic, the forty-year history of *Public Hygiene in Taiwan* (*TSKE* 1939). This report, a summary of numerous studies conducted by the public hygiene section of the police affairs department and a continuation of similar, previous reports, is a prime example for the paternalistic approach of the Japanese colonizers vis-á-vis the so-called 'islanders' of Taiwan. Throughout the report, the original population of Taiwan is usually labeled *hondōjin* (people of this island), a category that comprises the Han-Chinese population as well as non-Chinese aborigines but excludes the Japanese living in Taiwan as well as other foreigners (*TSKE* 1939, 12). The report emphasizes the benign influence of the efforts to improve the livelihood of the 'islanders' by demonstrating not only the overall population growth but also the decline in mortality from infectious diseases and the overall improvement of health and sanitation. This was achieved through the island-wide establishment of fifty-five clinics, ten laboratories, and two harbor quarantine stations to consequently detect and prevent the spread of infectious diseases (*TSKE* 1939, 93). To staff these institutional representations of modern Japanese medicine, a medical education system had started with a first medical school in 1899 and eventually resulted in the establishment of a full-fledged medical faculty of the Taipei Imperial University with an adjacent university hospital. The 1937 statistic lists the number of all staff members in one column, but the list of students distinguishes between Japanese students and 'islander' students. The absence of the distinction between Japanese and 'islanders' in the staff column is a strong indicator that all staff members were Japanese, especially since the distinction between Japanese and 'islander' was a constituting element in the administration of the school. A case in point is the yearly admission quota of the medical school of Taipei Imperial University. The overall quota was set at forty students, but instead of selecting all applicants along the same criteria, twenty places were reserved for Japanese students, and the other twenty places earmarked for 'islander' students. Thus, when in the 1937 intake 259 'islanders' and fifty-six Japanese applied for their respective twenty places, the mechanism of othering the non-Japanese students into another category than the Japanese students significantly reduced their chances for admission to the medical school vis-á-vis the Japanese applicants. The graduates of the medical faculty were supposed to replace the traditional healers and adherents to traditional Chinese medicine, which was dismissed as superstition by the new Japanese medical establishment (*TSKE* 1939, 43; Liu 2009, 97–104).

A considerable part of the hygiene report is devoted to the various infectious diseases that plagued the island. Cholera, the disease that had accompanied the opening of Japanese ports to foreign merchants in the late 1850s, broke out only three times in Taiwan's colonial era (1902, 1912, and 1919–1920), but its high mortality rate of 82 to 67 percent in these three waves made the disease a dreaded killer. Based on the Japanese experience with the pivotal role of ports for the spread of diseases, one of the first measures of the colonial administration in its fight against the spread of epidemics like cholera beyond ports was the establishment of a quarantine regime for the five major harbors of the island, which was modelled on the framework introduced for Japanese harbors with health inspectors, quarantine stations, and isolation hospitals. Thus, the island was equipped with sluices or locks to keep the germs out, which outsiders were bringing in, predominantly from the Chinese mainland (*TSKE* 1939, 92–4, appendix p. 4).

The introduction of modern hygiene in Taiwan thus came first and foremost in form of institutions like clinics, laboratories, quarantine stations, and sanitary police that worked according to Japanese principles of modernity. These institutions patronized the 'islanders' and discriminated against Taiwanese medical staff and students (Liu 2009, 134–9). Even the germs were othered as coming from China.

## The Bubonic Plague as the Litmus Test of Japanese Disease Control in Taiwan

One very dangerous germ circulating in the region in the early twentieth century caused the plague, which was called the 'Hongkong disease' in Taiwan since it supposedly had come to the island in the late nineteenth century via the port of Hongkong. Strict quarantine and a massive campaign to eradicate the disease on the island resulted in comparatively low numbers of deaths in the first two decades of the twentieth century and only a minimal number of infections after the end of the last big outbreak in 1917 (*TSKE* 1939, appendix 5). The plague is an interesting example to illustrate the mechanisms of othering in the realm of disease control. In the last decade of the nineteenth and the first decade of the twentieth century, several large outbreaks plagued the island with mortality rates around 80 percent. Outbreaks of the bubonic plague had occurred from the late eighteenth century onwards in southwest China from where the disease moved eastwards to reach Hongkong in 1894, from which it spread to all major seaports in the world. Tracing the plague in Chinese historical sources is not easy since the sources recorded diseases according to symptoms (that can be similar for a variety of diseases), used locally different names for diseases, or generically spoke of 'epidemics' without naming the disease. The fact that the plague was sometimes called the "rat epidemic," however, helps to follow its path to Hongkong from where it travelled to Taiwan (Benedict 1988, 108–9). Whereas a typical traditional Chinese medical practitioner in Southeast China explained the plague as caused by vapor (*qi*) that rose from the ground, affecting rats first because of their closeness to the ground and recommended fresh air as disease prevention as well as herbal treatment for the disease (137–8), the colonial government of Taiwan relied on the expertise of Japanese bacteriologists for combating the disease. Their actions were informed by germ theory and the conviction that Japanese medical researchers were at the forefront of international science since Japanese bacteriologist Shibasaburō Kitasato (1853–1931), a former student of Robert Koch, had gained an international reputation as co-discoverer, together with Alexandre Yersin (1863–1943), of the infectious agent of the bubonic plague in Hongkong during the outbreak of 1894 (Echenberg 2002, 437). Thus, the colonial government followed the recommendation of the bacteriological experts to detect cases of the plague as early as possible and isolate the patients. The compilation of the forty-year history of *Public Hygiene in Taiwan* proudly reports the success of the measures taken to eradicate the plague:

> Since 1901 ... the elimination of rats has been the basis of our disease control. Through the promotion of rat-proof houses and the improvement of neighborhood [sanitation], attempts are made to eradicate the plague, *in areas where the epidemic is particularly severe, entire villages were razed and burned.*

As a result, since 1918 there has been no trace of the plague. (*TSKE* 1939, 94; translated by the author with emphasis added)

The word "village" in this passage refers to rural settlements of indigenous people. The majority of the Japanese population lived in urban areas. As no colonial administrator would have ordered the scorching of Japanese dwelling in the name of disease control, reporting the eradication of entire indigenous villages as an adequate countermeasure against the plague shows a high degree of thoughtless othering of the 'islanders.' On the same page, the history of *Public Hygiene in Taiwan* reports with equal indifference the "construction of germ control camps" for those infected with typhus. A more benign countermeasure against the plague had been implemented in 1901 in form of an inoculation program that was, however, controversial, and short-lived. It was first introduced in an experimental form in six local communities and military compounds. Despite its initial success, it was not rolled out for the whole island, because this was seen as too costly. Liu cites the Sanitary Police's conviction as the main reason for its discontinuation, namely that, as a disease coming from 'unhealthy' China, the plague's spread was the result of the 'filthy' habits of the locals. Instead of wasting money on inoculation, they argued, the locals should learn to keep themselves and their environment clean (Liu 2009, 92).

The embodiment of filth as the breeding ground for disease was the rat, the elimination of rats the basis of disease control. Thus, in the beginning the colonial government even encouraged the killing of rats by paying some money for rodents delivered to the authorities—until some clever people started raising rats to collect the reward, and the scheme was discontinued in the first decade of the twentieth century (Liu 2009, 90). The forty-year history of *Public Hygiene on Taiwan*, compiled decades after the last major outbreak of the plague between 1914 and 1917 on the island, however, reports that in 1938:

[T]he plague, just like cholera, is not yet fully eradicated on the island. It is prevented from entering from outside the island by a port quarantine as well as the prohibition to import rags, old cotton, old clothes, old paper, etc., from Shanghai and other ports in China…. A large number of rats are bought up each year in each region to be tested for plague pathogens, just in case. In 1938, 311,262 rats were caught, of which 39,175 were examined for bacteria; all were germ-free. (*TSKE* 1939, 94; translated by the author)

*Figure 3: Poster from the* Anti-Plague Campaign in Taiwan 1916.
*(Taihokushū keisatsubu 1926.) Reprinted with the permission from the
National Taiwan University Library.*

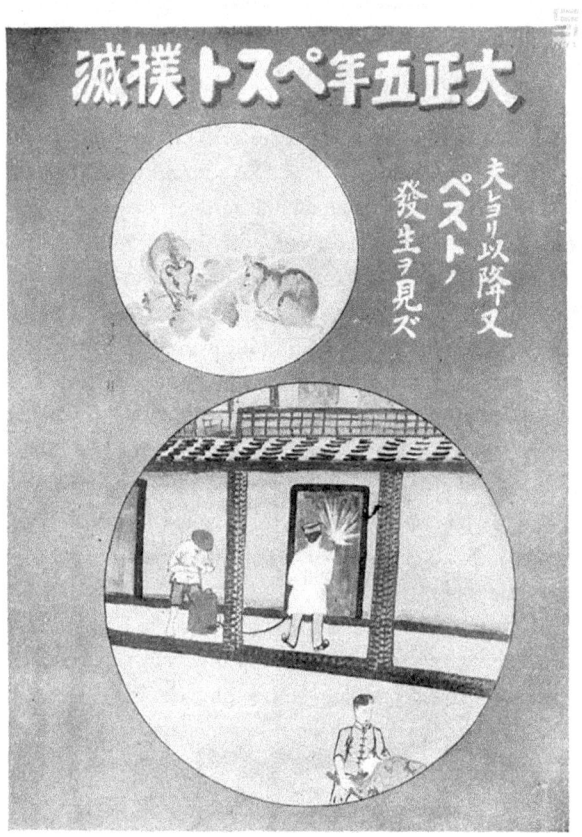

圖像來源：國立臺灣大學圖書館
Holding Institution: National Taiwan University Library
(TM_04_03_0014)

A propaganda poster from the last major outbreak of the plague 1914–1917
prominently features the culprit—the rat—and calls for the total eradication of
the plague. A drawing at the bottom of the poster shows a presumably Japanese
sanitary policeman in his professional Western outfit disinfecting the dwelling
of a plague victim that is being carried away in the foreground. His two local
helpers are dressed in a traditional Chinese outfit that does not protect them
as well from infection as does the medical garb of the sanitary officer. The fact

that the language on the poster is Japanese, just like the visual language, reveals the arrogance of the colonial administration that take language proficiency for granted for those educated enough to also understand the etiology of the disease and thus able to support the plague eradication campaign.

## Othering Through Sanitation

The Japanese colonial administration of Taiwan is often credited with the improvement of the living conditions on the island. Investment in public health and education made the population healthier and better educated, and life expectancy rose dramatically, thanks in part to the colonial government's fight against infectious diseases (Morgan and Liu 2007, 1016). Apart from the abovementioned direct countermeasures against the import and spread of infectious diseases as well as the creation of the medical infrastructure to treat the sick and educate medical practitioners in Western medicine, Japan's colonial health policy led also to the creation of sanitary infrastructure like clean water supplies and sewer systems. However, as Liu argues, this infrastructure was primarily installed in urban areas where the Japanese population congregated or in Japanese-owned plantation areas, and the positive health effects of these measures were mostly enjoyed by the colonizers (2009, 76). Campaigns to improve hygiene conditions in the countryside, where the Chinese population was less educated, had a rather basic character with suggestions for regulating drainage as well as education about parasites. The 'islanders' were usually portrayed as ignorant about the importance of cleanliness to avoid the spread of infectious diseases. A case in point is the chapter about water supply in the sanitation section of *Public Hygiene in Taiwan* which blames "unhygienic habits" for outbreaks of waterborne diseases after elaborating on overflowing sewers after torrential rainfall instead of addressing poverty as a possible reason for the derelict state of the sewage system of the average Taiwanese dwelling. Unhygienic *habits* [emphasis added] in discarding sewage, feces, and garbage are subsequently named as health hazards for the 'islanders.' The report also classifies the dwelling of the 'islanders' as unsuitable in its "all Chinese architecture" for modern sanitary standards. To combat the unhygienic habits, the "Major Cleaning Act" of November 1905 required "the entire island" to conduct major house cleanings twice a year, one in March and one in September, where not only the entire house but also wells and sewers had to be cleaned out, and special attention had to be devoted to the eradication of parasites and rodents

(*TSKE* 1939: 76–80). The ongoing existence of the "Major Cleaning Act" through-out the colonial period and its still being mentioned in the 1939 report on *Public Hygiene in Taiwan* show, however, that the colonizers did not trust the 'islanders' to integrate the spring- and autumn-cleanings as a useful habit once they experienced its benefit.

## Conclusion

After Japan's surrender at the end of the Second World War, the majority of the Japanese population in Taiwan was repatriated, although not all Japanese left the island immediately. Among those who remained was Toshirō Ōda (1893–1989), who resigned as the dean of Taipei Imperial University's Medical School in 1945 but held his professorship until 1947 when he returned to Japan (Liu 2009, 11). He is one of the colonizers whose contribution to the modernization of the island was appreciated. However, the appreciation of the achievements of Japanese colonial medicine should not disguise the fact that this success was achieved in a framework where mechanisms of othering were used to regulate the access to power. The device used was the newly developed concept of hygienic modernity. Japanese elites used a term traditionally connected to the individual preservation of health through taking care of one's body and redefined it as the embodiment of modern habits of cleanliness and health preservation through scientific knowledge about the transmission of infectious diseases. The colonial administration used a narrative in which those who understood and practiced modern hygiene justified their membership in the club of so-called civilized nations. In the logic of this narrative, the Others who procrastinated in the premodern worldview of traditional Chinese medicine and explained diseases like cholera or the plague through miasma or bad air, and had no idea about modern standards of cleanliness, had to be led into the modern era by the Japanese colonial administration of Taiwan.

## Works Cited

Arnold, David. 1993. *Colonizing the Body: State Medicine and Epidemic Disease in Nineteenth Century India*. Berkeley: University of California Press.
Bartholomew, James R. 1993. "Modern Science in Japan: Comparative Perspectives." *Journal of World History* 4, no. 1 (Spring): 101–16.

Beasley, William G. 1991. *Japanese Imperialism 1894–1945*. Oxford: Clarendon Press.

Benedict, Carol. 1988. "Bubonic Plague in Nineteenth-Century China." *Modern China* 14, no. 2 (April): 107–55.

Boyle, Edward. 2016. "Imperial Practice and the Making of Modern Japan's Territory: Towards a Reconsideration of Empire's Boundaries." *Geographical Review of Japan Series B* 88, no. 2: 66–79.

Echenberg, Myron. 2002. "Pestis Redux: The Initial Years of the Third Bubonic Plague Pandemic, 1894–1901." *Journal of World History* 13, no. 2 (Fall): 429–49.

Fukuda, Mahito. 1994. "Public Health in Modern Japan: From Regimen to Hygiene." In *The History of Public Health and the Modern State*, edited by Dorothy Porter, 385–402. Amsterdam: GA Rodopi.

GHS Index: Global Health Security Index. 2023. https://www.ghsindex.org/. Last Accessed September 20, 2023.

Gramlich-Oka, Bettina. 2009. "The Body Economic: Japan's Cholera Epidemic of 1858 in Popular Discourse." *East Asian Science, Technology, and Medicine* 30: 32–73.

Hée, Nadine. 2012. *Imperiales Wissen und koloniale Gewalt: Japans Herrschaft in Taiwan 1895–1945 (Imperial Knowledge and Colonial Violence: Japan's Rule in Taiwan, 1895–1945)*. Frankfurt: Campus Verlag.

———. 2014. "Taiwan under Japanese Rule: Showpiece of a Model Colony? Historiographical Tendencies in Narrating Colonialism." *History Compass*: 1–10.

Hirano, Katsuya, Lorenzo Veracini, and Toulouse-Antonin Roy. 2018. "Vanishing Natives and Taiwan's Settler-Colonial Unconsciousness." *Critical Asian Studies* 50, no. 2: 196–218. doi.org/10.1080/14672715.2018.1443019.

Jannetta, Ann B. 2007. *The Vaccinators: Smallpox, Medical Knowledge, and the 'Opening' of Japan*. Stanford: Stanford University Press.

———. 2009. "Jennerian Vaccination and the Creation of a National Public Health Agenda in Japan, 1850–1900." *Bulletin of the History of Medicine* 83: 125–40.

Johnston, William. 2019. "Cholera and the Environment in Nineteenth-Century Japan." *Cross-Currents: East Asian History and Culture Review* 30: 9–34. http://cross-currents.berkeley.edu/issue-30/johnston.

Joshi, Jayant S., and Rajesh Tewari. 2003. "Public Health and Sanitation in the Nineteenth Century Japan." *Proceedings of the Indian History Congress* 64: 1259–71.

Katz, Paul R. 1996. "Germs of Disaster: The Impact of Epidemics on the Japanese Military Campaigns in Taiwan, 1874 and 1895." *Annales de démographie historique*: 195–220.

Kitaoka, Shinichi. 2021. *Gotō Shinpei, Statesman of Vision: Research, Public Health, and Development*. Translated by Iain Arthy. Tokyo: Japan Publishing Industry Foundation for Culture.

Liu, Michael Shiyung. 2009. *Prescribing Colonization: The Role of Medical Practices and Policies in Japan-Ruled Taiwan, 1895–1945*. Ann Arbor: Association for Asian Studies.

———. 2011."An Overview of Public Health Development in Japan-Ruled Taiwan." In *Death at the Opposite Ends of the Eurasian Continent: Mortality Trends in Taiwan and the Netherlands 1850–1945*, edited by Theo Engelen, John R. Shepherd, and Wen-shan Yang, 165–81. Amsterdam: Amsterdam University Press.

Moon, M. Jae, Kohei Suzuki, Tae In Park, and Kentaro Sakuwa. 2021. "A Comparative Study of COVID-19 Responses in South Korea and Japan: Political Nexus Triad and Policy Responses." *International Review of Administrative Science* 87, no. 3: 651–71.

Morgan, Stephen L., and Michael Shiyung Liu. 2007. "Was Japanese Colonialism Good for the Welfare of Taiwanese? Stature and the Standard of Living." *The China Quarterly* 192, (December): 990–1017.

Myers, Ramon H., and Mark R. Peattie. 1984. *The Japanese Colonial Empire, 1895–1945*. Princeton: Princeton University Press.

Nomura, Akihiro. 1999. "Shokuminchi ni okeru kindaiteki tōchi ni kan suru shakaigaku: Gotō Shinpei no Taiwan tōchi o megutte" (Sociology of Modern Colonial Rule: Shinpei Gotō's Rule in Taiwan). *Kyoto Journal of Sociology* 7: 1–24.

Ozaki, Kōji. 2016. "Sensai Nagayo: Pioneer of Hygienic Modernity or Heir to Legacies from the Premodern Era?" *Otemae Daigaku Ronshū* 17: 61–88.

Peattie, Mark R. 1984. "Japanese Attitudes Towards Colonialism, 1895–1945." In *The Japanese Colonial Empire, 1895–1945*, edited by Ramon H. Myers and Mark R. Peattie, 80–127. Princeton: Princeton University Press.

Rogaski, Ruth. 2014. *Hygienic Modernity: Meaning of Health and Disease in Treaty Port China*. Berkeley: University of California Press.

Rubinstein, Murray A., ed. 2007. *Taiwan: A New History*. Armonk: M.E. Sharpe.

Said, Edward W. 1978. *Orientalism*. New York: Pantheon.

Scherer, Anke. 2019. "'Unreinheit' als Mechanismus der Ausgrenzung der 'Schmutzigen' und 'Nicht-Menschen' in der Edo-Zeit ('Impurity' as a Mechanism of Exclusion of the 'Dirty' and 'Non-Humans' in the Edo Period)." In *Outcasts in Japans Vormoderne: Mechanismen der Segregation in der Edo-Zeit (Outcasts in Premodern Japan: Mechanisms of Segregation in the Edo Period)*, edited by Stephan Köhn and Chantal Weber. 29–43. Wiesbaden: Harrassowitz Verlag.

Taihokushū keisatsubu (Taibei Provincial Police Department) (ed.). 1926. Taihokushū keisatsu eisei tenrankai shashinchō (Taibei Police Public Hygiene Exhibition Photobook). Taibei: Taihokushū keisatsubu.

Trambaiolo, Daniel. 2013. "Native and Foreign in Tokugawa Medicine." *The Journal of Japanese Studies* 39, no. 2 (Summer): 299–324.

———. 2014. "Vaccination and the Politics of Medical Knowledge in Nineteenth-Century Japan." *Bulletin of the History of Medicine* 88, no. 3 (Fall): 431–56.

TSKE (Taiwan sōtokufu keimukyoku eiseika) [Public Hygiene Section of the Police Affairs Department of the Governor-General of Taiwan]. 1939. Taiwan no eisei (Public Hygiene in Taiwan). Taibei: Taiwan sōtokufu keimukyoku eiseika.

Yamamoto, Shunichi. 1982. *Nihon korera-shi (The History of Cholera in Japan)*. Tokyo: Tokyo University Press.

# 5. Fear of Contagion: Epistemology of Boundaries and Politics of Emotions in (Post)Colonial Development Discourses

*Claudia Jahnel*

This article outlines strategies of othering in the context of COVID-19 from the perspective of postcolonial development studies. COVID-19 has reactivated stereotypes that have shaped the development discourse, including its sub-discourse on global health, since colonial times. The figure of the Other as a danger to one's own health and—historically directly linked to this—as a danger to national security occupies a central position here. Characteristic of the narratives of this discourse is, on the one hand, the high emotional charge that focuses on the stranger and intruder as a narrative of fear. This politics of emotion contributes to the legitimization of policies of border demarcation, resulting in a return of space and national territory. On the other hand, the narrative of the infectious, isolating and thus criminalized stranger perpetuates the idea of the superiority of Western industrialized nations, including their health systems and medical developments: "Europeans contrasted their own medicine and public health, symbolizing rationality and modernity, with putatively superstitious and primitive indigenous medical beliefs, which they denigrated and sought to eliminate as part of the larger 'civilizing mission' of colonialism" (King 2002, 765).

Postcolonial development studies combine two research perspectives that are in clear tension with each other. While development research is oriented towards implementable solutions to problems and the "transformation of society along universal guiding principles," postcolonial studies unmask these very guiding principles as Eurocentric constructs (Ziai 2010; my translation). "One field"—postcolonial theory—therefore "begins where the other [development studies] refuses to look." (Sylvester 1999, 704). The postcolonial critique of development research and discourse begins with the understanding of 'de-

velopment' itself and the normalization and thus normativity of a Western understanding of development, because

> [t]he metrices of development that delimit the 'developed' and 'developing'
> were established in the post-second world period [which] despite the suc-
> cess of decolonization movements across the world ... was rooted in existing
> colonial power structures. [Its] system of privilege is often referred to as in-
> visible power or assets, as it often remains unacknowledged and obscured
> by institutions and structures. (Padmanabhan et al. 2021, 212)

Postcolonial critique thus questions the epistemological assumptions of the
development discourse that continuously perpetuate inequalities. On the
other hand, development research also points out the deficits of postcolonial
theory. These lie primarily in the "intellectualisation" (Sylvester 1999, 703) and
"hyperaesthetisation" of this "actually anti-hegemonic theorising" (Castro-
Varela and Dhawan 2015, 340; my translation). Hence, while "development
studies does not tend to listen to subalterns ... postcolonial studies does not
tend to concern itself with whether the subaltern is eating" (Sylvester 1999,
703).

The discussion of COVID-19 from the perspective of postcolonial development studies takes account of these mutual points of criticism. For the pandemic is one of those challenges "within which colonial institutions and ideas
are being moulded into the disparate cultural and socio-economic practices
which define our contemporary 'globality'" (Loomba 1998, 257). The COVID-19
discourse reflects powerful colonial ideas and institutions; they break open and
swirl around like in a kaleidoscope, yet cannot be easily isolated, but appear
in ever new constellations. Unlike initial assessments of the "corona society"
(Volkmer and Werner 2020; my translation) and the "world after the pandemic"
(Kortmann and Schulze 2020; my translation), which judge the Corona crisis
as a historical break in history, as an "epochal threshold" or as an expression
of a "dead end" into which modernity has fallen (Adloff 2020, 149; my translation), the continuities predominate from the perspective of postcolonial development studies. One might even ask whether the rhetoric of crisis is not an
expression of a Euro-/North American-centric perspective. For it seems to be
shaped by precisely that teleological and evolutionist understanding of development whose claim to universal validity postcolonial theory is challenging.

This becomes paradigmatically clear when Vera King, for example, speaks
of the "shattering of cultural patterns": "The figure of the eternal departure as

a cultural pattern of processing and defending against transience has … become cracked on different levels: morally or normatively, practically in life and thus also in the psychological and psychosocial sense" (2020, 123–4; my translation). Whose cultural pattern are we talking about here? Can the "figure of eternal departure" be culturally universalized as a "defense against transience"? From a postcolonial perspective, the teleological-evolutionist understanding of modernity that the talk of the "figure of eternal departure" seems to imply obscures the view of the possibility of thinking other futures. The COVID-19 "crisis" and the shattering of this Eurocentric model of time therefore also allows for other concepts of future-making to come into sight (Appadurai 2013). I will elaborate these aspects in the last paragraph of this article.

In 2023, there seems to be little left—on a global-economic level—of the fundamental "shattering" observed by Vera King, which would have led us to expect equally fundamental changes in cultural and social patterns. Even euphoric claims such as Slavoj Žižek's (2020) that the virus would deal a decisive blow to global capitalism and finally make room for international and interpersonal solidarity must, from today's perspective, be seen as a transitional phenomenon. Has the virus not rather unmasked the sheer egoism that will continue to shape the economy and social coexistence in the future? In any case, vaccine nationalism in the competition for the development of vaccines against the virus and the failure of the solidarity-based idea of a global 'procurement community' initiated by the WHO and originally also by COVAX (COVID-19 Vaccines Global Access) demonstrates the persistence of the logic of monopolization of power and knowledge in the Global North and thus the return to 'business as usual.' The question 'Health security for whom?' can thus be answered very clearly: primarily for the Global North.

Postcolonial development studies focus on stories that illustrate that COVID-19 has aggravated global as well as intersectional inequalities (Obeng-Odoom 2020; Blume 2022). For example, COVID-19 had a disproportionate impact on the culture of African Americans who were not allowed to mourn their deceased (Mitchell 2020). Numerous studies also show the higher vulnerability of Black Americans. A paradigmatic example of this is the story of the Black American physician, Dr. Susan Moore, who died from COVID-19 "two weeks after she had shared publicly how a White physician had not taken her physical health complaints seriously" (Blume 2022, 58). Postcolonial development studies examines the overt racism evident in examples like these in light of and as a consequence of colonial logics and practices that have become deeply inscribed in the body.

## The Danger of Contagion: Epistemology of Delineation

The contemporary processes of globalization have torn down many of the boundaries of the colonial world. Along with the common celebrations of the unbounded flows in our new global village, one can still sense also an anxiety about increased contact and a certain nostalgia for colonialist hygiene. The dark side of the consciousness of globalization is the fear of contagion. If we break down global boundaries and open universal contact in our global village, how will we prevent the spread of disease and corruption? ... The age of globalization is the age of contagion. (Hardt and Negri 2003, 136)

A look back to March 2020:[1] COVID-19 escalates fear of infection. Face masks and disinfectants are sold out. Grocery shops have surrounded their cash registers with plexiglas and used tape on the floor to mark the distances customers should keep from each other—to minimize the risk of infection. Posters like *Stay Safe—Save Lives—Stay Home* are omnipresent. Solidarity means keeping your distance. An isolationist imperative prevails (Žižek 2020). Border closures are once again seen as an act of sovereignty (Han 2020) and as an attempt to reactivate the interest in immunologizing the state and nation once associated with the territorial state of the nineteenth century. Because a territorially and nationally reorganized state seemed to promise "a bounded geographical space that provides a basis for material resources, political power, and common allegiance" (Maier 2000, 816).

In the midst of the comprehensive borderlessness of globalization as well as of a "borderless permissive society" (Han 2020; my translation) that does not stop at physical borders in the various variants of the exploitation of others and of oneself in the existing performance society, COVID-19 has made borders highly acute again. In an era marked by digitalization and virtuality, geographical space is back—in all its vulnerability, which is most evident in the very effort to immunologically seal it off. The enemy is not—or at least not primarily—another state power or ideology, as in the case of the Cold War or 9/11. The enemy is a pandemic, a virus that nevertheless mobilizes the entire arsenal of war rhetoric from "crisis team" to "security risk" and "combat" as well as the deployment of *Bundeswehr* reservists. This comparison of the pandemic to war

---

1   My deliberations refer back to an article that I wrote in March 2020: Jahnel, Claudia. 2020. "Entwicklungszusammenarbeit in Zeiten von Covid-19 – postkoloniale Relektüre." In *Jahrbuch für Christliche Sozialwissenschaft Bd. 61/2020: Postkolonialismus und Theologische Ethik*, edited by Marianne Heimbach, 21–31. Münster: Aschendorff.

seems to counter the anxiety caused by COVID-19 and to meet the hope that the pandemic can be controlled and defeated (Lehtinen and Brunila 2021).

The fear of contagion on the one hand and a politics and epistemology of boundary-setting and delineation on the other (King 2002) have not only been present since COVID-19, but, as the quotation from Michael Hardt and Antonio Negri illustrates, accompany the ongoing globalization. In the Corona 'crisis,' however, this scheme of stimulus—fear of contagion—and reaction—drawing of boundaries—has taken on a concrete, existentially threatening and highly emotionalized appearance. For the individual and the individual's behavior in cases of a pandemic, a certain limitation is certainly sensible. However, the stimulus-response schema must be critically questioned if it serves to legitimize boundaries and distances to the Other, as was and is often the case in colonial and postcolonial contact as well as in development work that emerged in the colonial and postcolonial context. From the beginning, the colonial Other was considered contagious and dangerous.

The French writer and doctor Louis-Ferdinand Céline portrays the Other in his famous colonial novel *Journey to the End of the Night* (1932): "These n\*\*\* are sick, they're perverts! You'll see ... Degenerate scum!" (1992, 142). Poor physical condition and moral decay thus go hand in hand and demand that the supposedly healthy and civilized European keeps a distance to the Other. What makes this 'disgusting society' so dangerous, however, is not lifelessness, but—on the contrary—its exuberant fullness of life: "What a horror for a hygienist! This disease that the colony lets loose is the lack of boundaries on life, an unlimited contagion" (Hardt and Negri 2003, 135)—then and now. In the words of Marlow, the protagonist of Josef Conrad's *Heart of Darkness* (1902): "But suddenly ... a whirl of black limbs, a mass of hands clapping, of feet stamping, of bodies swaying, of eyes rolling .... The prehistoric man was cursing us, praying to us, welcoming us—who could tell? We ... glided past like phantoms, wondering and secretly appalled as sane men would be before an enthusiastic outbreak in a madhouse" (1991, 23–4, 57). For the sterile-hygienic order of the "healthy" European, this "lack of boundaries on life" is dangerous (Hardt and Negri 2003, 148). Protection for the explorer, the European soldier, settler, trader or employee of the colonial administration is provided by borders and fences—also around mission stations (Jahnel 2015, 187–8), rules that keep the Other at a distance such as the prohibition of mixed marriages, and a dichotomizing ideology that constructs a clear difference to the self by depicting the Other as underdeveloped, uncivilized, raw or heathen.

## International Development and Health Politics and Economic Security

The logic—'fear of the Other, therefore boundary setting'—remains un-changed. Only the patterns of justification and strategies shift and sometimes conceal the violence of boundary setting behind the appearance of charity, especially in development policy and international health policy. Hence, the concern for the health of the indigenous population, which became the focus of colonial health policy in Germany at the time of the colonial empire, was not based on humanitarian-egalitarian motives. Rather, economic, techni-cal, medical, military, political, and religious-cultural interests of leading countries in Europe were the crucial driving factor.

A central motive of colonial health policy was the preservation and in-crease of the labor force, because growth and health of the population in the colonies—especially women's health—represented the central condition for the economic growth of the colonizing nations. The influential state physician Ludwig Külz (1875–1938), for example, saw the crucial "task of the tropical hygienist" to "profitably utilise" the "living capital stock" in the "service of the colonial economy" and to increase population density (qtd. in Dübgen 2010, 430; my translation). From the middle of the twentieth century, however, overpopulation in the 'Third World' was seen not only as a cause of poverty and health for the countries of the Global South, but also as a security risk for the industrialized nations. International health and development policy therefore introduced birth control programs from the 1960s onwards. The United Nations Population Fund (UNFPA; formerly United Nations Fund for Population Activities), for example, supported anti-natalist programs in the 1970s, such as India's sterilization camps under Indira Ghandi (Deuser 2010, 436). So again, like in the colonial era, women formed the central target group for development and health programs. In this context, they were mostly con-ceptualized and othered as a uniformly stereotypical quantity—as the "Third World woman" (Mohanty 1988; my translation). This is still true of the most recent approach in the field of development cooperations, the empowerment approach, which is associated with the International Conference on Popula-tion and Development (ICPD) in Cairo in 1994, often presented as a 'paradigm shift.' However, this approach still has an "antinatalist bias" (Schultz 2006). Again, it does not, as Patricia Deuser analyses, "lead to a dismissal of colonial racist and culturalist assumptions about the Other, but again reproduces 'women in developing countries' as a homogeneous group who have internalized the potential to overcome inequality, this time qua gender" (Deuser 2010, 448; my translation).

## International Development and Health Politics, Political Security and Colonial Amnesia

International health policy and the narrative of security—predominantly for the conquerors and colonial powers—are closely linked. As early as the nine-teenth century, international agreements were decided on quarantine regula-tions to limit the spread of cholera, plague and yellow fever in international trade. The World Health Organization (WHO) continued this policy with the fight against polio, smallpox, tuberculosis, malaria or sleeping sickness.

The narrative of political security is thereby closely linked to the centuries-old imagination that contagion, sickness and death are caused by the stranger; as Susan Sontag states:

> One feature of the usual script for plague: the disease invariably comes from somewhere else. The names for syphilis, when it began its epidemic sweep through Europe in the last decade of the fifteenth century, are an exemplary illustration of the need to make a dreaded disease foreign. It was 'the French pox' to the English, 'morbus germanicus' to the Parisians, the 'Naples sick-ness' to the Florentines, the 'Chinese disease' to the Japanese. But what may seem a joke about the inevitability of chauvinism reveals a more important truth: that there is a link between imagining diseases and imagining foreign-ness. (1989, 135)

Illness and epidemics are therefore a challenge for foreign and security poli-tics. In the recent past, the stimulus-response logic of fear, border demarca-tion, foreign and security policy is probably nowhere more striking than in migration and refugee policy. In her essay "Invasion, Infection, Invisibility," Francesca Falk (2010) has shown how in the "iconology of illegitimate immigra-tion" refugees are repeatedly associated with dangerous diseases and the risk of infection. The depiction of emaciated refugees supported by helpers wear-ing protective masks, or of overcrowded and therefore epidemic-suspicious refugee boats not only feeds racist fears of contact. It also activates strate-gies of immunization that, with their medical, political-national and economic promises, mark the beginning of modernity (Esposito 2004).

A blind spot—Arthur Blume calls this even a "colonial amnesia and forgotten horrors" (2022, x)—is the fact that the diseases introduced by the conquerors—above all influenza, measles, smallpox, and typhus—cost the lives of millions of people in the conquered territories (Livi-Bacci 2006; Bianchine and Russo 1992). Epidemics, thus, "played a critical role in colonization, weakening Indigenous resistance and killing millions through the Columbian exchange" (Blume 2022, 1).

## International Development and Health Politics and Competitive Capability

International health policy was, after all, also about international scientific competitiveness and hegemony. Virologists like Robert Koch or later the tropical physician August Hauer, who developed drugs against diseases like cholera, malaria and sleeping sickness, had no qualms about conducting dehumanizing experiments on the indigenous population (Besser 2002). European exceptionalism once legitimized unethical measures, just as Trumpian exceptionalism recently could consider the purchase of exclusive rights to a vaccination against COVID-19 ethically unproblematic (Butler 2020).

The practice of drawing boundaries also shapes the binary distinction between Western advanced medicine and 'primitive,' 'superstitious' traditional medicine, which is a cantus firmus of Western development work. The "horror" or the "abject" (Kristeva 1982) to be repelled is no longer the "n***," as in Céline, but "only" the medicine of the "n***." This demarcation becomes the basis of legitimacy for the spread of Western medicine and development aid to the Global South. The humanitarian appearance that development aid thus gains at the same time conceals not only geopolitical self-interests, but also the epistemic violence with which non-Western knowledge and belief systems are destroyed and local agency is marginalized by Western experts. Even the new headings of international health care, 'global health' or 'health in One World,' only seem to break this binary discourse logic. They suggest a reorganization of North-South relations and a common global interest but conceal unjust structures. Talk of the "One World" is in fact, as postcolonial development researcher Aram Ziai criticizes as "cognitively incapacitating, analytically insufficient and politically consequential": The term "One World" "deprives individuals of the possibility of a self-determined articulation of their own interest, does not differentiate between the extremely unequal socio-economic conditions of the actors and the related situations of interest, and distracts from privileges and conflicts of interest in the emphasis on common interests and necessary cooperation" (2006, 129; my translation).

## International Mission and Epidemics: Health as Religious Task

In the context of mission, health becomes a religious task, because caring for the sick and dying is interpreted as an act of charity and self-sacrifice to which Christianity—like other religions—obliges believers (Höpflinger 2016). Along with education and preaching, health care was one of the three central pillars of mission. Visually, these were reflected in the construction of hospitals, schools, and churches.

In religiously motivated development and health care, too, epidemics in general are the 'diseases of the Others.' They are observed, studied, and cured, but always from a distance. Characteristic of the context of religious health care, however, is a "schema of pain," according to which the observers are requested to let themselves be affected by the suffering of the Other and to take on the pain of the Other in the imagination (Thomas 2021; my translation). Reports from the mission field and photos served not least the purpose that the observers back home perceived how the caring sisters in their self-sacrifice and devotion become more and more like the serving love of Christ (Gause 2021, 116).

One contagious disease that received special attention in the context of mission in the nineteenth century was leprosy. The photographic representation of leprosy was, as Richard Hölzl analyzes, characterized by an "aesthetics of suffering" in the sense of Susan Sontag's famous book-length essay *Regarding the Pain of Others*: That is, the mediation of distant suffering was intended to trigger an aestheticizing effect in the viewer and, not least, a willingness to donate money to the mission work (Hölzl 2016, 95; my translation). Here, in the practice of religious health care as well as in its visual mediation, the emphasis is less on promoting a fear of contagion than on stimulating a compassionate interpretation of suffering controlled by 'aesthetic regimes' and learned through cultural viewing habits. Hölzl therefore rightly understands leprosy not only as a "boundary disease," "by means of which the boundaries of a society are negotiated and determined," but also as an "entangled disease," i.e. a "disease with a transnational history of entanglement" (Hölzl 2016, 98; my translation). This special attention that Christian mission paid to leprosy is certainly due, first, to the visibility of leprosy as a skin disease. Yet, secondly, the fact that leprosy is already mentioned in biblical stories of illness and healing and has a rich representation in Christian art marked leprosy as a very peculiar epidemic disease and furthered a discourse of similarity that mobilized the affects and emotions in a special way (Grön 1930). The sick and suffering Other is, however, also in these entangled dynamic processes and despite all the agency that Hölzl sees shimmering through in the documents 'between the lines,' the product of a powerful, hierarchizing othering and the object of a 'white charity.'

## Aesthetic Regimes of the Development Discourse: Othering Dynamics via Hypervisibility

The uncanny aspect of the Corona 'crisis,' which fueled diffuse fears, was the invisibility of the virus, especially in the first year of the pandemic: neither is the 'enemy'—the virus—visible, nor is it possible to see in advance who already has and is spreading the virus. This invisibility correlates with the invisibility of the victims: the sick are not 'shown'—for good reasons of preserving the dignity of the individual and personal rights. Only anonymous coffins—but some of them in mass photographs—make the effectiveness of the virus visible. This is true for large parts of the Global North.

This invisibility is contrasted by the hypervisibilization of COVID-19 victims from the Global South, be it African Americans in the USA, or victims of other epidemics and infectious diseases that have spread mainly in the Global South. In addition to the already mentioned leprosy, these include the more recent epidemics Ebola in Liberia in 2014 and Congo in 2019 and cholera. Similar to civil wars in African countries or the so-called refugee crisis, the spread of diseases and epidemics in the Global South is dominated by a flood of photographic images which often convey the impression of poverty and underdevelopment, of the aforementioned "lack of boundaries" and of huge crowds of people which already in principle are an obstacle to compliance for hygienic protection measures. Victims of COVID-19 and other epidemics in the Global South are thus much more exposed to the public gaze that objectifies them, in contrast to the victims in the Global North who are not shown. But it is precisely this visualization that plays the central role in the success of the 'white charity' that aid organizations invoke. For, according to this logic, the visualization of the victims mobilizes the viewer's emotions of consternation and compassion—misericordia—as well as the financial willingness to help (Kiesel and Bendix 2010). This visual representation of the Other has numerous pre-decessors in missionary photography and in the photographic documentation of medical and anthropological research (Ratschiller and Weichlein 2016).

The visibilization of the effects that COVID-19 had in the Global North, on the contrary, is limited either to posters giving instructions on hygiene or to photos of medical personnel in protective suits, their faces covered and hidden behind masks, asking the population to stay at home. This inequality of representation underlines all the more the processes of othering that accompany the display of the bodies of the Other. The visibly suffering body of the Other marks a need for help, a lack of agency and a lack of sovereignty. Under the othering, distancing gaze of the scientist or the benefactor, the body of the Other is objectified, disenchanted, degraded. At the same time, the visualization of the body of the Other activates a victim-savior schema that calls the helpers into the subject position and makes them benefactors, if not saviors. The heroic figures of the Corona 'crisis' are the medical professionals, the virologists and hygiene experts, although they also often turned out to be the scapegoats and conspirators. The role of victims in the Global North remains visually largely unoccupied. It seems to contradict the social imagination of the West to be presented as vulnerable. The fear of infection, however, is diverted to fantasies of technical feasibility and of one's own, European or North American, immunity and invulnerability.

The development and global health discourse, with its rhetoric of war on the one hand and its visual representation of the vulnerable Others onto whom one's own vulnerability is projected on the other hand, evokes points of contact with Judith Butler's political philosophy and her exhortations to be mindful of one's own vulnerability:

> Mindfulness of this vulnerability can become the basis of claims for non-military political solutions, just as denial of this vulnerability through a fantasy of mastery (an institutionalized fantasy of mastery) can fuel the instruments of war. We cannot, however, will away this vulnerability. We must attend to it, even abide by it, we begin to think about what politics might be implied by staying with the thought of corporeal vulnerability itself, a situation in which we can be vanquished or lose others. Is there something to be learned about the geopolitical distribution of corporeal vulnerability from our own brief and devastating exposure to this condition? (2004, 29)

Slavoj Žižek (2020) has characterized this awareness of one's own vulnerability the "most disturbing lesson" of the COVID-19 crisis: "Human beings are much less sovereign than they think .... They must be able to endure this without going crazy" (my translation). This insight is not new, and it is repeated in the Corona 'crisis' in numerous references to the unifying vulnerability of being human. But people's own vulnerability has obviously been forgotten or repressed in times of colonial health as well as in (post)colonial development 'aid.'

Exceptions confirm the rule. One of these exceptions is the declaration "Heil und Heilung" (Salvation and Healing) (DifäM 2000), which emerged from a groundbreaking international ecumenical conference in 1964, known as "Tübingen 1," initiated by the World Council of Churches and the Lutheran World Federation. "Heil und Heilung" not only constructively integrates the insight into the limited sovereignty of human beings into questions of development cooperation, but the declaration also anticipates many aspects of postcolonial perspectives in its programmatic presentation of Christian development cooperation in the field of health. Amid the departure of former colonized territories for independence, the participants of "Tübingen 1" recalled principles of the Christian mission of healing and development. According to the declaration, central to Christian self-understanding and Christian social ethics is the tension between inaccessibility and responsibility. Healing is not only the result of human medical action, but also—from a religious point of view—a gift and sign of the dawn of the kingdom of God. Moreover, healing is not limited to physical processes, but is a relational event. This means that healing includes the healing of social relationships and standing up for each other in solidarity. Therefore, healing is not only the task of experts, but a mandate for the whole of society, locally, globally, transnationally, and decentrally, because it is about the vulnerability of the one world. This understanding of development and health puts into question—at least in theory—processes of othering that are prevalent in the logic of developmental aid and global health discourses.

## Time and the Other: Multiple Temporalities

One crucial point of postcolonial critique regarding the hegemonic discourse on development is its conceptualization of time and especially of future. I have already mentioned that the dominating teleological and evolutionist model of time has prevented the perception of other concepts of future making. Furthermore, the dominating Eurocentric concept of time has furthered the idea of the superiority of the so-called West which presented and continues to present itself as more advanced than the Other. One legacy of colonialism and of colonial ethnography is that the Other was and is projected into another, more primitive time zone and has been denied coevalness. This non-simultaneity is expressed not only in the explicit reference to a different temporal order (Fabian 1983). Rather, it manifests itself throughout the field of ethnographic writing and has produced a 'temporal lexicon,' a lexicon of temporally coded terms imbued with interests and power. Terms such as 'savagery,' 'kinship' or 'primitive'—the key term of the temporalizing discourse—are therefore not 'innocent' descriptions but have connotations of temporal value: they suggest a 'historically earlier' time in connection with moral, aesthetic, and political implications. Georg Hegel's conception of Africa as a continent without development and history is probably one of the peak points in this discourse on time and the Other and demonstrates the epistemic violence and the polemic inherent in it. In his *Philosophy of History*, Hegel writes that Africa "is no historical part of the World; it has no movement or development to exhibit. ... What we properly understand by Africa is the Unhistorical, Undeveloped Spirit, still involved in the conditions of mere nature" ([1899] 1956, 99). Crises have always given rise to predictions and scenarios for the future, ranging from the imagination and anticipation of a more solidary society to apocalyptic visions. COVID-19, thus, can and has been taken as an opportunity for a fresh look at alternative concepts of time and future, and—as the imaginations of the future turn future into the present—COVID-19 has provided a space to reflect and negotiate visions of life and to bring to the fore visions that have been silenced and marginalized.

The term 'future' has been appearing frequently in German and international development cooperation for some years now. In 2014, the Federal Ministry for Economic Cooperation and Development (BMZ) published the "Zukunftscharta—EINEWELT, unsere Verantwortung" (Future Charter: ONE WORLD—Our Responsibility; my translation), which focuses on the question of the sustainability of development: how can development be advanced in such a way that it sustainably secures the economic, ecological, and social future for all? Development is no longer considered only a 'problem' of the Global South. With climate change and international political and religious conflicts—as well as pandemics—the future of all people is at stake and requires a 'great transformation'; this means: a comprehensive rethinking of the global, local and individual use of resources.

These new perspectives are remarkable, because for a long time the discourse on development and modernity did not grant a future to the countries of the Global South, as e.g. Felwine Sarr states:

> In positing, right from the outset, that modernity is a teleological concept, the reflection becomes inherently flawed. But we posit this flaw within modernity as a necessary occurrence within the emergence of societies, and we do this by considering it from an evolutionary perspective. Furthermore, instead of thinking the social dynamics under way in the manner in which they present themselves and then extracting meaning from them, we will content ourselves, on one hand, to trace the presence or absence of the signs of modernity within the real of African societies, and on the other hand, to posit as signposts its philosophical principles (the apologia of the new, reason as the foundation of social organization) and the institutional forms it provides for itself. As such, in simply measuring the distance separating various African societies, we condemn ourselves to experiencing the pangs of comparison, perpetually thinking of ourselves like some sort of straggler, always striving to catch up in order to gain a place in the various rankings that constantly remind us how we've fallen behind. This leads the becoming subject to fall prey to the good-student complex. (2019, 20–1)

COVID-19 was accompanied by an interruption of this teleology of imagined futures and the notion of catch-up development which perceives the present state of the industrial nations as the normative future for nations of the Global South. Detlef Müller-Mahn and Eric Kioko observe that "[t]he external origin of the disease reinvigorated resentment against foreign influence in general, and against Western remedies and Eurocentric visions of development in particular" (2022, 28–9). Furthermore, "[w]hat had previously been hailed as gateways to modernization and prosperity—airports, roads, and trade corridors—became entry points for a potentially fatal threat" (29). COVID-19 reveals the uncertainty of the futures that were and are anticipated—and promised—by the development discourse.

It is in this context that demands to decolonize the future are starting to be heard—even in the Global North. Against, for instance, the Afro-pessimist stereotype that perceives Africa as continent of catastrophes and as 'no-future place,' academic scholars (e.g. Mbembe 2015; Sarr 2019), as well as artists and Afrofuturist movies (*Neptune Frost* 2021, *Black Panther* 2018, etc.) are insisting on the need to stop mimicking Western concepts and to "dare to reinvent the Future" of African traditions (Sarr 2019, 91). These demands are not a form of nativist romanticization of the African past (Mbembe 2001) but rather a call for epistemic freedom (Ndlovu-Gatsheni 2018). "Can Africans create African futures within a modern world system structured by global coloniality?" (Ndlovu-Gatsheni 2014, 181). Sabelo Ndlovo-Gatsheni's question corresponds with the concluding statement of the postcolonial scholars Castro-Varela and Nitika Dhawan: "However, it still seems possible for us to make other futures conceivable"—with the help of postcolonial theory (2015, 340; my translation).

COVID-19 has revived stereotypes of the Other and has exacerbated inequalities and aggravated injustices. It thus continues to be a test case for development cooperation and global politics which are in urgent need of critical postcolonial and socio-ethical reappraisal. But, at least in theory and in some parts of cultural and development studies, it has also increased the insight into global vulnerability—contrary to the claim of 'white supremacy'—and it has signalled an emerging awareness of a polyphony of futures.

## Works Cited

Adloff, Frank. 2020. "Zeit, Angst und (k)ein Ende der Hybris." In *Die Corona-Gesellschaft*, edited by Michael Volkmer and Karin Werner, 143–54. Bielefeld: transcript. https://doi.org/10.14361/9783839454329-015.

African Studies Association. (2016) 2017. "ASA 2016 Abiola Lecture with Achille Mbembe." Delivered by Achille Mbembe, uploaded February 3, 2017. YouTube, https://www.youtube.com/watch?v=J6p8pUU_VH0.

Appadurai, Arjun. 2013. *The Future as Cultural Fact: Essays on the Global Condition.* London: Verso.

Besser, Stephan. 2002. "Germanin. Pharmazeutische Signaturen des deutschen (Post)Kolonialismus." In *Kolonialismus als Kultur. Literatur, Medien, Wissenschaft in der deutschen Gründerzeit des Fremden*, edited by Alexander Honold and Oliver Simons, 167–95. Tübingen: A. Francke.

Bianchine, Peter J., and Thomas A. Russo. 1992. "The Role of Epidemic Infectious Diseases in the Discovery of America." *Allergy and Asthma Proceedings* 13, no. 5: 225–32. https://doi. org/10.2500/108854192778817040.

Blume, Arthur W. 2022. *Colonialism and the COVID-19 Pandemic: Perspectives from Indigenous Psychology.* International and Cultural Psychology Series. Cham: Springer. https://doi.org/10.1007/978-3-030-92825-4.

Butler, Judith. 2004. *Precarious Life: The Powers of Mourning and Violence.* London: Verso.

———. 2020. "Capitalism Has Its Limits." *Verso*. March 30, 2020. https://www
.versobooks.com/blogs/4603-capitalism-has-its-limits.

Castro-Varela, María do Mar, and Nikita Dhawan. 2015. *Postkoloniale Theorie: Eine kritische Einführung*. Bielefeld: transcript.

Céline, Louis-Ferdinand. (1932) 1988. *Journey to the End of the Night*. Translated
by Ralph Manheim. London: John Calder.

Conrad, Joseph. (1902) 1991. *Heart of Darkness*. New York: Harper and Brothers.

Deuser, Patricia. 2010. "Genderspezifische Entwicklungspolitiken und Bevöl-
kerungsdiskurse: Das Konzept der 'Sexuellen Reproduktiven Gesundheit
und Rechte' aus postkolonialer Perspektive." *Peripherie* 30, no. 120: 427–51.

Deutsches Institut für Ärztliche Mission (DifäM), ed. 2000. *Die vernachlässig-
ten Dimensionen: Auseinandersetzungen mit Gesundheit und Heilung im ökume-
nischen Prozess*. Studienheft 3. Tübingen: DifäM.

Dübgen, Franziska. 2010. "'Respect the Poor'? Postkoloniale Perspektiven auf
Armut." *Peripherie* 30, no. 120: 452–77.

Esposito, Roberto. 2004. *Immunitas: Schutz und Negation des Lebens*. Translated
by Sabine Schulz. Berlin: Diaphanes.

Fabian, Johannes. 1983. *Time and the Other: How Anthropology Makes its Object*.
New York: Columbia University Press.

Falk, Francesca. 2010. "Invasion, Infection, Invisibility: An Iconology of Ille-
galized Immigration." In *Images of Illegalized Immigration: Towards a Critical
Iconology of Politics*, edited by Christine Bischoff, Francesca Falk, and Sylvia
Kafehsy, 83–100. Bielefeld: transcript.

Gause, Ute. 2021. "Kranke auf die Ewigkeit ausrichten: Leiden, Behinderung
und Tod und ihre Transzendierung in Bethel im 19. Jahrhundert." In *Dem
Schmerz begegnen: Theologische Deutungen*, edited by Katharina Greschat and
Claudia Jahnel, 115–28. Bielefeld: transcript.

Grön, Kristian. 1930. "Lepra in Literatur und Kunst." In vol. A/10/2 of *Handbuch
der Haut- und Geschlechtskrankheiten*, edited by Josef Jadassohn, 806–42.
Berlin: Springer.

Han, Byang-Chul. 2020. "Wir dürfen die Vernunft nicht dem Virus überlassen."
*Welt*. March 23, 2020. https://www.welt.de/kultur/plus206681771/Byung-C
hul-Han-zu-Corona-Vernunft-nicht-dem-Virus-ueberlassen.html.

Hardt, Michael, and Antonio Negri. 2003. *Empire: Die neue Weltordnung*. Frankfurt: Campus.

Hegel, Georg Wilhelm Friedrich. (1899) 1956. *The Philosophy of History*. New York:
Cover Books.

Hölzl, Richard. 2016. "Lepra als entangled disease. Leidende afrikanische Körper in Medien und Praxis der katholischen Mission in Ostafrika 1911–1945." In *Der schwarze Körper als Missionsgebiet: Medizin, Ethnologie, Theologie in Afrika und Europa 1880–1960*, edited by Linda Ratschiller and Siegfried Weichlein, 95–121. Köln: Böhlau.

Höpflinger, Anna-Katharina. 2016. "Zwischen Repräsentation und Regulierung: Körper als Aushandlungsorte für Weltanschauungen." In *Der schwarze Körper als Missionsgebiet: Medizin, Ethnologie, Theologie in Afrika und Europa 1880–1960*, edited by Linda Ratschiller and Siegfried Weichlein, 175–87. Köln: Böhlau.

Jahnel, Claudia. 2015. *Interkulturelle Theologie und Kulturwissenschaft: Untersucht am Beispiel afrikanischer Theologie*. Stuttgart: Kohlhammer.

Kiesel, Timo, and Daniel Bendix. 2010. "White Charity: Eine postkoloniale, rassismuskritische Analyse der entwicklungspolitischen Plakatwerbung in Deutschland." *Peripherie* 30, no. 120: 482–95.

King, Nicholas B. 2002. "Security, Disease, Commerce: Ideologies of Postcolonial Global Health." *Social Studies of Science* 32, no. 4/6 (October–December): 763–89.

King, Vera. 2020. "Ewiger Aufbruch oder Einbruch einer Illusion: Muster der Verarbeitung von Vergänglichkeit vor und in der Folge von 'Corona.'" In *Jenseits von Corona: Unsere Welt nach der Pandemie—Perspektiven aus der Wissenschaft*, edited by Bernd Kortmann and Günther G. Schulze, 117–26. Bielefeld: transcript.

Kortmann, Bernd, and Günther G. Schulze, eds. 2020. *Jenseits von Corona: Unsere Welt nach der Pandemie—Perspektiven aus der Wissenschaft*. Bielefeld: transcript. https://doi.org/10.14361/9783839455173.

Kristeva, Julia. 1982. *Powers of Horror: An Essay on Abjection*. Translated by Leon S. Roudiez. New York: Columbia University Press.

Lehtinen, Mattias, and Tuukka Brunila. 2021. "A Political Ontology of the Pandemic: Sovereign Power and the Management of Affects through the Political Ontology of War." *Frontiers in Political Science* 3 (July). https://www.frontiersin.org/articles/10.3389/fpos.2021.674076/full.

Livi-Bacci, Massimo. 2006. "The Depopulation of Hispanic America after the Conquest." *Population and Development Review* 32, no. 2: 199–232. https://www.jstor.org/stable/20058872.

Loomba, Anita. 1998. *Colonialism/Postcolonialism*. London: Routledge.

Maier, Charles. 2000. "Consigning the Twentieth Century to History: Alternative Narratives for the Modern Era." *American Historical Review* 105, no. 3 (March): 807–31.

Mbembe, Achille. 2001. "Ways of Seeing: Beyond the New Nativism. Introduction." *African Studies Review* 44, no. 2 (September): 1–14.

———. 2015. "Decolonizing Knowledge and the Question of the Archive." Last Accessed February 2023. https://wiser.wits.ac.za/system/files/Achille%20 Mbembe%20-%20Decolonizing%20Knowledge%20and%20the%20Questi on%20of%20the%20Archive.pdf.

Mitchell, Elise A. 2020. "'If Bitterness Were a Whetstone': On Grief, History, and COVID-19." *Black Perspectives*. April 23, 2020. https://www.aaihs.org/if -bitterness-were-a-whetstone-on-grief-history-and-covid-19/.

Mohanty, Chandra Talpade. 1988. "Aus westlicher Sicht: Feministische Theorie und koloniale Diskurse." *Beiträge zur feministischen Theorie und Praxis* 11: 149–62.

Müller-Mahn, Detlef, and Eric Kioko. 2022. "COVID-19, Disrupted Futures, and Challenges for African Studies." In *African Futures*, edited by Clemens Greiner, Steven van Wolputte, and Michael Bollig, 28–35. Leiden: Brill. htt ps://doi.org/10.1163/9789004471641_004.

Ndlovu-Gatsheni, Sabelo J. 2014. "Global Coloniality and the Challenges of Creating African Futures." *Strategic Review for Southern Africa* 36, no. 2: 181–202.

———. 2018. *Epistemic Freedom in Africa: Deprovincialization and Decolonization.* New York: Routledge.

Obeng-Odoom, Franklin. 2020. "COVID-19, Inequality, and Social Stratification in Africa." *African Review of Economics and Finance* 12, no. 1: 3–37.

Padmanabhan, Martina, Samia Dinkelaker, Mareike Hoffmann, Dimas Laksmana, Siti Maimunah, Elena Rudakova, Enid Still, and Friederike Trotier. 2021. "Principles of Critical Development Studies: A Minifesto." *ASIEN* 160/161 (July–October): 210–20. https://www.researchgate.net/profile/Ma rtina-Padmanabhan/publication/365852803_Principles_of_Critical_Devel opment_Studies_A_Minifesto/links/63887b677d9b40514e044064/Principl es-of-Critical-Development-Studies-A-Minifesto.pdf?origin=publication _detail.

Ratschiller, Linda, and Siegfried Weichlein, eds. 2016. *Der schwarze Körper als Missionsgebiet: Medizin, Ethnologie und Theologie in Afrika und Europa 1880–1960.* Köln: Böhlau.

Sarr, Felwine. 2019. *Afrotopia.* Translated by Drew S. Burk and Sarah Jones-Boardman. Minneapolis: University of Minnesota Press.

Schultz, Susanne. 2006. *Hegemonie—Gouvernementalität—Biomacht: Reproduktive Risiken und die Transformation internationaler Bevölkerungspolitik.* Münster: Westfälisches Dampfboot.

Sontag, Susan. 1989. *Illness as Metaphor and AIDS and Its Metaphors.* New York: Picador.

———. 2004. *Regarding the Pain of Others.* London: Penguin.

Sylvester, Christine. 1999. "Development Studies and Postcolonial Studies: Disparate Tales of the 'Third World.'" *Third World Quarterly* 20, no. 4: 703–21.

Thomas, Günter. 2021. "Schmerzen beobachten: Techniken, Funktionen und faszinierende Objekte." In *Dem Schmerz begegnen: Theologische Deutungen*, edited by Katharina Greschat and Claudia Jahnel, 19–33. Bielefeld: transcript.

Volkmer, Michael, and Karin Werner, eds. 2020. *Die Corona-Gesellschaft: Analysen zur Lage und Perspektiven für die Zukunft.* Bielefeld: transcript. https://doi .org/10.14361/9783839454329.

Ziai, Aram. 2006. *Zwischen Global Governance und Post-Development: Entwicklungspolitik aus diskursanalytischer Perspektive.* Münster: Westfälisches Dampfboot.

———. 2010. "Postkoloniale Perspektiven auf 'Entwicklung.'" *Peripherie* 120, no. 30: 399–426.

Žižek, Slavoj. 2020. "Der Mensch wird nicht mehr derselbe gewesen sein: Das ist die Lektion, die das Coronavirus für uns bereithält." *NZZ.* March 13, 2020. https://www.nzz.ch/feuilleton/coronavirus-der-mensch-wird-nie-mehr-derselbe-gewesen-sein-ld.1546253.

"Zukunftscharta—EINE WELT, unsere Verantwortung." 2014. *Bundesministerium für wirtschaftliche Zusammenarbeit und Entwicklung (BMZ).* Last Accessed March 29, 2020. https://www.bmz.de/de/mediathek/publikationen/reihe n/infobroschueren_flyer/infobroschueren/Materialie250_zukunftscharta .pdf.

# 6. The Other as Conspirator: Historical Roots of COVID-19 Conspiracy Theories

*Martin Tschiggerl*

Throughout the COVID-19 pandemic, many studies have been published that analyze the spread and emergence of conspiracy theories in times of health crisis and around health policies (e.g. Bruns, Harrington, and Hurcombe 2020; Uscinski et al. 2020; Shahsavari et al. 2020; Hotez 2020; Douglas 2021; Pummerer et al. 2020; Ullah et al. 2021; Pummerer, Winter, and Sassenberg 2022). Especially in the first two years of the pandemic, the analysis of these conspiracy theories lacked a historical classification and contextualization. As a result, ahistorical and predominantly present-oriented explanatory models were used to analyze these theories, ignoring the fact that recent conspiracy theories surrounding health policies and pandemics have historical roots, the origins of which can reach back for more than several centuries. This is slowly beginning to change, however, as an anthology edited by Michael Butter and Peter Knight (2023) shows. This article is another first preliminary study of such historical roots. At its core is a comparison of conspiracy theories that emerged in the context of COVID-19 with historical conspiracy theories that circulated about smallpox in the late nineteenth and first half of the twentieth century. In both cases, vaccination is a central reference point within these theories. As previous studies have shown, vaccinations play an important role within many of the present-day conspiracy theories around health policies (Leask and Chapman 2002; Kata 2010; Kata 2012; Nan and Daily 2015; Dredze, Broniatowski, and Hilyard 2016; Safford, Hamilton, and Whitmore 2017; Sharma et al. 2017; Smith and Graham 2017; Bricker and Justice 2019; Hotez 2020). No other health policy measure is as successful but at the same time as controversial as vaccinations, as they are a health policy measure that affects everyone and has therefore been and still is widely discussed by society (Thießen 2017).

In this article, I analyze and compare radical opponents of vaccination in the German-speaking world in the late nineteenth, early twentieth and twenti-

first centuries, exploring the role that conspiracy theories play in their arguments. 'Radical' in this context means that they reject vaccination in its entirety, not just compulsory vaccination and that this rejection is combined with
conspiracy theories and anti-science attitudes. As I will also show, othering is
a central aspect of these conspiracy theories. In German-speaking countries,
anti-Semitic conspiracy theories are a recurring narrative.

Following Michael Butter and others, I define conspiracy theories as complex narratives that explain historical or contemporary phenomena as the result of a conspiratorial plan by a particular group or individuals (2018; Butter and Knight 2021; Douglas, Sutton, and Cichocka 2017). They are cohesive,
mono-causal, and self-referential theories that regard all explanatory models
lying outside their own narrative as part of the very conspiracy they seek to
uncover. In the logic of conspiracy theories, nothing happens by chance, but
they create connections and causalities where none would be found without
them (Barkun 2013). According to Geoffrey Cubitt (1989), conspiracy theories
assume an intentional conspiracy to achieve a specific plan, they are characterized by a dualistic worldview that clearly divides the world into good and
evil, and they make an occultist distinction between a visible world and a secret one that needs to be uncovered. Conspiracy narratives attempt to reduce
complexity, but in the process, they can themselves take on decidedly complex
forms. For the people who believe in them, they can take on almost ideological functions, that is, they can shape their fundamental view of the world,
habitus, and everyday practices (Pfahl-Traughber 2015). As Robbie M. Sutton
and Karen M. Douglas showed, at least for recent historical moments and the
present, conspiracy beliefs can be observed across the political spectrum; however, these beliefs are particularly prevalent in political extremism, with right-
wing extremist ideologies being somewhat more prone to them than left-wing
extremists (2020). Studies of current conspiracy theories suggest that ideolog-
ical-predisposing conditions play a central role in the formation and belief of
conspiracy theories (Smallpage, Enders, and Uscinski 2017; Miller, Saunders,
and Farhart 2016). In this regard, Roland Imhoff and Martin Bruder also refer to a "conspiracy mindset" as the tendency, when someone believes in one
conspiracy theory, to also believe in other conspiracy theories (2014).

In the context of conspiracy beliefs, health policy and politics per se,
so-called meta-conspiracy theories or super-conspiracy theories are rampant.
These grand theories represent a connecting link between different conspiracy narratives and, as such, are particularly powerful since they function as
ideological reality generators sui generis for those who believe in them. Anti-

Semitism, for example, represents a classic form of meta-conspiracy theory (Pfahl-Traughber 1993). From the second half of the nineteenth century on-wards, the conspiracy theory component of anti-Semitism consisted primarily of the idea of an international Jewish world conspiracy. Part of this imagined conspiracy was both Jewish capitalism, which German anti-Semites ciphered as the "Golden International," and Jewish communism/socialism (Simon-sen 2020, 360). In this article, I analyze the connections between a belief in conspiracy theories and radical rejections of vaccination from a historical per-spective and illustrate how strongly this rejection is linked to a simultaneous othering of imagined conspirators.

Conspiracy theories create an 'us' and a 'them' in two respects: First, by distinguishing between the victims of the imagined conspiracy and the per-petrators, that is, the conspirators. Here, there is a clear division into 'good' and 'evil,' with clearly distributed roles, whereby a distinction can be made whether the imagined 'evil'—that is, the conspirators—are already in power or are trying to gain power through the conspiracy. Butter refers to conspiracies from above versus conspiracies from below (2018, 29–33). Current conspir-acy theories around COVID-19 suggest almost exclusively conspiracies from above, while historical theories from the nineteenth century tend to claim conspiracies from below, such as a secret plot by Jews to gain world domina-tion, for example. Of course, this also strongly depends on where in the social hierarchy the conspiracy theory believer is located: political elites are likelier to imagine conspiracies from below, while marginalized persons are likelier to see conspiracies from above. A second form of othering then concerns those who 'know' about the conspiracy—the enlightened ones, so to speak—and those who know nothing about it and perhaps even mock the enlightened ones, often called "sheep" by conspiracy theory believers (Van Prooijen 2019, 319). This is also a self-exaltation of those who believe in conspiracy theories; they themselves are the chosen ones who know the truth. On a meta-level, one may, of course, also note that the classification 'conspiracy theory' is a form of othering as well. At least in the last fifty years, this label has also functioned as delegitimization and exclusion from discourse—anyone who is called a conspiracy theorist is generally no longer taken seriously (Bratich 2008). 'Conspiracy theory' in this article represents a term of analysis based on the classification in this introduction.

In my analysis, I draw an arc from the nineteenth to the twenty-first cen-turies to show, with the help of selected examples, the linkage of radical anti-vaccination attitudes with conspiracy theories and, in particular, anti-Semitic narratives. My sources are statements published by central representatives of the anti-vaccination movement. Due to the broad historical perspective, I can only present a few selected representatives. For the nineteenth century, I focus on the Berlin politician Paul Förster, chairman of the *Deutscher Bund der Impfgegner*, for the twentieth century, on representatives of the National Socialist 'New German Medicine' and for the twenty-first century, I analyze two central figures of the German-speaking *Querdenker* scene, Attila Hildmann (Germany) and Martin Rutter (Austria).

These are selected representatives of a strong combination of anti-vaccination attitudes and ideological resentment. To illustrate this, I analyze statements made by these exponents to show how they fuse elements of conspiracy theory and anti-Semitic topoi. For this purpose, I have analyzed Förster's publications on the one hand and the Telegram channels of Hildmann and Rutter on the other. Methodologically, I used a qualitative discourse analysis, the results of which I summarize in this study.

## Anti-Vaccination Movements and Anti-Semitism in History

In 1874, the German Reichstag passed the so-called *Reichsimpfgesetz* (Imperial Vaccination Act), which, following the English model, created a legal obligation to have children immunized against smallpox.[1] Already in Great Britain, which in the last third of the nineteenth century was considered a model for compulsory vaccination, the introduction of compulsory vaccination was accompanied by fierce protests (Durbach 2005). References to the situation in Great Britain and repeated attempts to network with the anti-vaccination movement were therefore a recurring motif of the German anti-vaccination movement (Thießen 2017, 37). However, the positions of the German opponents of vaccination differed from those of the English due to the sometimes strong overlaps with anti-Semitic and *völkisch* milieus (Nebe, Schwanke, and Groß 2021). The *völkisch* movement attained political importance from the last third of the nineteenth century, both in the German Empire and in the Habsburg Empire. It was based at its core on a racist understanding of the concept of *Volk*, which

---

1   On the opponents of the *Reichsimpfgesetz* in Germany, see Eberhard Wolff's "Medizinkritik der Impfgegner im Spannungsfeld zwischen Lebenswelt und Wissenschaftsorientierung" (1996).

was linked to the desire for a homogeneous nation and racist ideas of superiority as well as Social Darwinist ideas of a survival of the fittest (Puschner,
Schmitz, and Ulbricht 2012).

There were two distinct groups opposing mandatory vaccinations in the
German Empire. On the one hand, there were mainly liberal-minded people
who did not reject vaccinations per se but the state's intervention in the individual bodies of its citizens. Hence, their criticism was directed at the obligation for vaccination. The second group of opponents of this law completely rejected vaccinations, not just the obligation to vaccinate. This second, very heterogeneous group, recruited from various alternative milieus, was united primarily by their radical and strict opposition to vaccination: homeopaths, animal rights activists, vegetarians, nudists or alternative medicine practitioners
(Wolff 1996).

Eugen Dühring, for example, claimed in his book *Die Judenfrage als Racen-,
Sitten- und Culturfrage*, published in 1881, that vaccinations were purely a
money-making scheme by Jewish doctors propagated in association with
Jewish publicists and Jewish politicians (19). The author thus insinuates a deliberate conspiracy to propagate vaccination that is part of an imagined Jewish
conspiracy. Dühring's pamphlet is considered one of the prototexts of a modern, racially legitimized anti-Semitism and, as such, represents a blueprint
for the anti-Semitism of the later National Socialists (Longerich 2021, 99–101).
This combination of hatred of Jews and rejection of vaccinations did not arise
in a vacuum but is part of a *völkisch* ideology that also manifests itself in
various alternative medical movements, which were decidedly conceived as a
countermovement to orthodox medicine and modern life. This is particularly
evident in the example of the Berlin grammar schoolteacher, publicist and
politician (Arthur) Paul Förster (Nebe, Schwanke, and Groß 2021). Förster was
not only a convinced anti-Semite, but also a radical opponent of vaccination.
As a member of the Reichstag, he agitated against compulsory vaccination; as
a publicist, he published inflammatory writings against Jews and campaigned
for animal protection and against vivisections. Förster was the founder of the
*Deutscher Bund der Impfgegner* and one of its most important spokesmen, as
well as a signatory of the *Antisemitenpetition* of 1880/81. As Julia Nebe, Enno
Schwanke and Dominik Groß have shown, Förster's anti-vaccine agitation is
strongly rooted in his anti-Semitic, *völkisch* ideology. This is based on the idea
that the German race and, in particular, German blood, must be protected
from Jewish influences. Vaccinations were seen as such a Jewish influence,
while at the same time, they were rejected as an intervention in natural life

that ran counter to a social-Darwinian understanding of nature. In his various writings, Förster is firmly opposed to "modern science," which he repeatedly describes as "superstition" and which would only distance humans further and further from nature (1900, 104, 153, 161, 246, 247; n.d.; my translation). The (in his opinion) Jewish-influenced scientific medicine and especially vaccinations are his clear enemies, which would weaken and ultimately destroy the German people (1900; 1906; 1907). He himself advocates a return to nature and natural ways of life through which a healthy and, above all, homogeneous ethnic body is to be preserved.

In his argumentation, Förster can be clearly located within the so-called *Lebensreform* movement, which began to appear in the middle of the nineteenth century as social reform initiatives for a more 'natural' way of life. Their representatives agitated against industrialization, urbanization and, to some extent, precisely against orthodox medicine. The German term *Schulmedizin* (school medicine), which is still used today, originated within this movement as a derogatory term for what they saw as unnatural scientific medicine (Eckart and Jütte 2007, 374–5). In particular, the *völkisch* parts of the *Lebensreform* movement provided an excellent environment for conspiracy narratives from the end of the nineteenth century and the beginning of the twentieth century onward. Jews represented a particularly and frequently used form of the Other in these imagined conspiracies, as they were seen as part of modern urban life and an imagined Other to the homogeneous German people (Longerich 2021, 151–4; Breuer 2005). In this context, Förster combined *völkisch*, anti-Semitic, life-reformist and naturopathic ideas—vaccinations are read as part of an artificial and modern, Jewish life and contrasted with a natural and traditional, German life.

Thus, it was only a relatively short distance from the negatively connoted *Schulmedizin* to the *verjudeten Schulmedizin*, which was set within certain currents of National Socialism as an imagined Other to a Germanic-set naturopathy. The strongly pronounced *völkisch* and racist thinking within different varieties of these movements enabled a seamless transition into the ideology of National Socialism. Leading elites of the *Nationalsozialistische Deutsche Arbeiterpartei* (NSDAP) and the NS state had a strong connection to naturopathic movements and combined their rejection of orthodox medicine with their radical anti-Semitism. On the part of the Nazi system, after the 'seizure of power,' there was an attempt to bundle these different movements under the common brackets of the *Neue Deutsche Heilkunde* and to give them a more 'scientific' approach (Bothe 1991; cf. Ernst 2001). Rudolf Hess, Deputy Führer of the NS-

DAP, was one of the most authoritative promoters of alternative medical movements within the Nazi elite. The *Rudolf-Hess-Krankenhaus* in Dresden endorsed the attempt to scientifically prove the efficacy of alternative medical practices such as homeopathy and to combine alternative approaches such as fasting, hydrotherapy, herbalism, or homeopathy with scientific ones. However, this scientific proof failed and the *Neue Deutsche Heilkunde* lost more and more of its significance from 1941 onwards, especially after Hess's flight to Great Britain (Ernst 2001; Lienert 1998). Besides Hess, Heinrich Himmler, *Reichsführer-SS*, was also a vehement anti-vaccinationist, as was Julius Streicher, founder and editor of *Der Stürmer*, who published anti-vaccination, anti-Semitic cartoons in *Der Stürmer* and supported the founding of another anti-vaccination magazine (Thießen 2017, 144–7). In their minds, vaccination was a sinister plot by Jewish doctors to poison the German people and stain their German blood. Even though the various anti-vaccination associations placed great hopes in the Nazi state, these very associations were banned in the course of the prohibition of any opposition and the *Gleichschaltung* of the state. Although the vaccination obligation was partially relaxed, the Nazi state also launched massive vaccination campaigns—after all, the outbreak of the war and the presence of millions of forced laborers in the Reich meant that the people, the army and especially the *Wehrkraft* had to be protected against infectious diseases (Thießen 2017, 144–7). Although the anti-vaccination radicals in the Nazi state thus suffered defeat despite the initial hopes and massive support of at least some of the Nazi elites, the alternative medical movements in particular were able to build on the successes of the interwar period and the institutional valorization of alternative medicine during the Nazi era after 1945. In particular, the various parts of the *Lebensreform* movement remained strongly rooted in Germany and Austria, and many of their ideological successors form the nucleus of the *Querdenker* protests in the present day (Frei and Nachtwey 2022).

## The *Querdenker*

In March 2020, both the German and Austrian governments felt compelled to take drastic measures to contain the novel coronavirus. Horror pictures from northern Italy, where the virus was rampant, dominated media coverage. Therefore, strong action by governments to protect their citizens seemed urgently needed. These governmental measures in some respects included massive constraints on public life and the individual freedom of citizens, such as contact restrictions and compulsory closures of shops, restaurants and virtually all public facilities. In short, public life came to a standstill for several weeks (Thießen 2021). In reaction, considerable resistance first formed on social media and subsequently on the streets of numerous major cities (Benz 2021). Already in March 2020, the first demonstrations against the aforementioned measures were announced in Germany and Austria. Out of this resistance emerged a protest movement commonly referred to as the *Querdenker*, or 'lateral thinkers.' This is an extremely heterogeneous movement that, at least at the beginning, encompassed a wide variety of social groups, subcultures and political camps. Based on a sociological study of the Corona protests, Nadine Frei and Oliver Nachtwey distinguish between four different milieus from which the protesters were recruited: the alternative milieu, the anthroposophical milieu, the Christian evangelical milieu, and a middle-class protest milieu (2021). Already in the first months of the protests, however, it became apparent that in both Germany and Austria, right-wing extremist individuals and organizations increasingly began to take the lead within the movement and to appropriate it for themselves, respectively, to use it as a platform (Thießen 2021, 139–43). From the outset, conspiracy theories formed an ideological and integrative framework that generated common ground within the *Querdenker* movement. From the beginning, these conspiracy theories revolved around the causes and the 'true' nature of the pandemic. Widespread conspiracy narratives explained the pandemic as a 'plandemic,' that is, a deliberately controlled event. Bill Gates, who had already been involved in global vaccination campaigns in the past, was imagined as a central actor and seen as one of the string pullers in the background (Butter 2021).

Anti-Semitic narratives played a central role in the German-language *Querdenker* movement from the very beginning (Wetzel 2021). Due to the social ostracism of open anti-Semitism in the German-speaking world after 1945, it is mainly the so-called camouflage anti-Semitism that appears in the context of the Corona protests. Camouflage means that anti-Semitic ideas are articulated without directly naming Jews as Jews (Rensmann 2008). This happens, for example, through the use of codes such as 'Rothschilds,' 'Rockefellers,' 'Ostküste,' 'Globalists,' or 'New World Order.' But even if the terminology has changed through the use of these codes, these conspiracy theories are part of a long tradition of anti-Semitic conspiracy theories in the German-speaking world in which Jews are imagined as evil Others and made responsible for imagined or actual problems (Salzborn 2021).

In this context, the radical QAnon conspiracy theory was able to gain a foothold in the German-speaking world. This conspiracy theory first appeared on the largely unmoderated US online message boards 4chan and 8chan in 2017 and gained noticeable momentum in Germany in the wake of the Corona protests (Keil 2022). The core of this theory is the belief in a secret, satanic power elite that imprisons children, tortures them, and uses their blood for secret rituals and as a rejuvenation serum. Within this theory, the enemy is primarily the political establishment in the USA, in particular the Democratic Party, and Donald J. Trump is presented as a kind of savior (Amarasingam and Argentino 2020). The QAnon theory is an extremely complex meta-conspiracy theory that combines and bundles different narratives. It builds on classical anti-Semitic myths that have been widespread in Europe since the Middle Ages. For example, the claim that Jews sacrifice children and abuse their blood for religious rituals (Butter and Knight 2021). The Corona pandemic led to an update of the theory by identifying COVID-19 as part of the secret world elite's plan to control, enslave and ultimately destroy the population. For believers in the theory, vaccinations are a central aspect of this secret and, above all, sinister plan.

Anti-vaccination sentiments played a central role within the *Querdenker* milieu from the beginning, along with the rejection of wearing protective masks months before vaccination against the coronavirus was even available. Nadine Frei, Robert Schäfer and Oliver Nachtwey attest to the *Querdenker* movement's high affinity for conspiracy theories and also note that, politically speaking, the movement tended to originate from the political left, but in the course of the pandemic, it has increasingly moved to the right (2021). Social media plays a central role in the networking and communication of the protest movement, with the messaging service Telegram being the most widely used medium of this kind (Holzer 2021). While other social media platforms such as Facebook, Twitter and YouTube have increasingly taken action against the dissemination of misinformation in recent years—not least due to government pressure—Telegram has not yet taken any steps in this direction. This is why many of the figureheads of the Corona protests run their own Telegram channels.

For Austria, the former right-wing politician Martin Rutter (BZÖ) is particularly noteworthy. Rutter acted as an organizer for demonstrations throughout Austria and runs several channels (Rutter n.d.). The most successful of these is "Impfschaden_D_AUT_CH," with around 77,000 members. On this channel, Rutter collects reports of alleged problems caused by the vaccination against COVID-19, such as severe diseases or even deaths and then uses these in his other channels to agitate against vaccination and other protective measures against the spread of the virus. Since June 2021, reports of tens of thousands of severe side effects with alleged thousands of deaths have been registered on this channel. Rutter publishes these reports as a "Vaccine Damage Archive" on his website, completely unchecked, under the title "Vaccination Kills" and passes them off as facts (n.d.; my translation). However, he also uses the group to advertise his other Telegram channels. In these other channels, he posts content that he has produced himself or shares content from relevant scene portals, such as the right-wing extreme Austrian news site "Aufi." A recurring motif is the conspiracy theory of the "Great Reset." This theory is based on the book *COVID-19: The Great Reset*, published by Klaus Schwab and Thierry Malleret, which calls for a reorganization of the world economy following the pandemic (2020). However, conspiracy theory reinterprets this initiative discussed at the World Economic Forum 2020 to the extent that the COVID-19 pandemic is understood as a planned event through which the world's economic elite wants to reshape the world according to their ideas (Birchall and Knight 2022). In his context, Rutter repeatedly uses the term "globalists," which must be understood as an anti-Semitic code (n.d.; my translation). This becomes particularly clear in a post from April 2020, in which Rutter published a photo showing the then Austrian Chancellor Sebastian Kurz (ÖVP) with George Soros and his son Alexander Soros with the comment "Freunderl, Globalisten und 'Corona Diktatoren' unter sich" (Friends, globalists and 'Corona dictators' among each other) (Rutter 2020; my translation). The philanthropist and billionaire Soros has repeatedly been the victim of anti-Semitic campaigns and hostility in recent years, especially in Austria, and serves here as a platform for the implicit assumption of a Jewish conspiracy (Hannig 2020). This is an example of camouflage anti-Semitism that functions without the explicit naming of Jews but relies on codes that are understood by the recipients. However, the example of one of the main figures in the German *Querdenker* movement, Attila Hildmann, shows how quickly a strongly coded anti-Semitism can turn into an open one.

Hildmann began his career as a restaurant owner and author of vegan cookbooks and gained prominence in Germany through a number of TV appearances. Since 2020, however, he has been known for his role in the *Querdenker* protests. Together with the likewise prominent singer, Xaiver Naidoo, he was one of the most radical voices in the markedly heterogeneous scene of this movement.[2] Hildmann was not only the organizer of some of the largest demonstrations in Berlin and their main speaker, but also runs his own Telegram channel, which at its most successful had around 120,000 members (Hildmann n.d.).[3] Meanwhile, Hildmann is wanted in Germany on an arrest warrant for incitement of the people and has probably absconded to Turkey ("Attila Hildmann" n.d.). The reason for this warrant is Hildmann's open anti-Semitic agitation, especially on his Telegram channel. Jews and an imagined Jewish world conspiracy play a central role in this channel. For him, the COVID-19 pandemic is a plot orchestrated by a Jewish world conspiracy in pursuit of a sinister agenda. An analysis of his Telegram channel shows that Attila Hildmann's content has become increasingly anti-Semitic over the course of the pandemic, even though he was already one of the most extreme voices in the first year of the pandemic. In 2020, Bill Gates, in particular, represented a central reference point in Attila Hildmann's theories. He was imagined as part of a global conspiracy, the New World Order, and was perceived as the central mastermind behind the fake Corona pandemic, which aimed to control or even destroy humanity through vaccination. Hildmann combines an anti-elitism often observed in conspiracy theories with the rejection of vaccination. Vaccinations are once again the central reference point—they are the instrument through which the elites operating in secret want to achieve their sinister plans. Bill Gates offers the ideal focal point for this; even before the COVID-19 pandemic, he was a popular bogeyman within conspiracy theories because of his commitment to global vaccination campaigns. Already at this early stage, Hildmann used strongly anti-Semitic codes, such as "Zionists," "Globalists" and "Rothschilds," but very rarely spoke directly of Jews (Tschiggerl 2023). This changed from 2021 on. From then on, Hildmann openly spoke of Jews and their alleged secret world conspiracy on his Telegram channel. He used the marker 'Jew' as a form of othering for virtually all his imagined enemies. In the course of this, for example, Angela Merkel and Bill Gates—neither of whom are Jewish—also became Jews. It is obvious that Hildmann relied on his followers' own anti-Semitism—for example, he claimed that all major vaccine

---

2    Unlike Hildmann, Naidoo has since apologized for his earlier remarks in a highly ac-claimed video and openly admitted to be a believing conspiracy theorist.

3    The Telegram channel was the target of several hacking attacks and was offline mul-tiple times. At the time of final editing of this article (1.4.2023), it was online, but not accessible from German cellular networks.

producers were run by Jews and relied on the fact that the attribution 'Jew' alone made it clear to his readers that they were pursuing evil intentions.

Hildmann and Rutter are both extreme examples within the *Querdenker* milieu. However, they are representative in that they have both been organizers of large demonstrations and run particularly wide-reaching Telegram channels. This also applies to Paul Förster. He, too, was one of the most radical voices within the German-speaking anti-vaccination movement of the late nineteenth and early twentieth centuries, but he, too, was one of the movement's figureheads as an association chairman and organizer of international anti-vaccination congresses. The main aim of this article has been to outline continuities in the ideological link between radical opposition to vaccination and conspiracy-theoretical anti-Semitism.

## Conclusion

This study has shown that within the so-called *Querdenker* movement, conspiracy theories are widespread, which repeatedly mobilize anti-Semitic topoi and practices of othering (Wetzel 2021). Although the propagators of these conspiracy theories, apart from their most radical representatives, such as Attila Hildmann, refrain from using the term 'Jews' directly, the use of code words such as "Globalists," "Rothschilds" or "New World Order" makes it clear who the real culprits in the pandemic are supposed to be. This is a camouflage anti-Semitism that works strongly with codes and tries to bypass the social ostracism of open anti-Semitism in the German-speaking world (Rensmann 2008). Thus, current conspiracy theories draw on historical ones and show clear parallels to conspiracy theories that can be traced back to the nineteenth century. Vaccinations are the key frame of reference, both in the present and in the past. After all, vaccinations are at the same time the most successful but also the most controversial health policy technique and have been strongly disputed since the beginning of their application. They have been particularly controversial when there has been public debate on the possibility of compulsory vaccination in acute pandemic situations. In this regard, the smallpox epidemics of the nineteenth and early twentieth centuries provide an excellent comparative framework for the Corona pandemic of the twenty-first century. This comparison reveals a long history of anti-science discourse within the various anti-vaccination movements, often accompanied by a high affinity for conspiracy theories. This can be understood as an expression of magical thinking that makes connections where none would be found without belief in conspiracy theories and that believes in a world beyond the visible – precisely the world of conspiracy and the secret machinations that pull the strings in the background. The radical rejection of vaccinations has often gone hand in hand with anti-modern resentment. Romantic notions of a 'natural body' and a 'back to nature' tendency represent important points of orientation as a counter-position to a medical science that is perceived as unnatural and thus rejected. However, the resulting conflicts must also be understood as a struggle for medical and social hegemony and the question who has power over people's health: the respective individuals, naturopathic 'healers,' scientific medicine or even the state apparatus? Conspiracy theories serve to impute evil intentions to others—be it 'science,' 'medicine' or 'the Jews'—and to legitimize one's own position. Especially, the focus on 'Jews'—no matter if they are named directly or addressed by code words—is a distinctive characteristic of the German-language anti-vaccination movement and its associated conspiracy theories. Here, one can clearly see the parallels between current debates about COVID-19 and historical debates about smallpox.

## Works Cited

Amarasingam, Amarnath, and Marc-André Argentino. 2020. "The QAnon Conspiracy Theory: A Security Threat in the Making." *CTC Sentinel* 13, no. 7 (July): 37–44. https://ctc.westpoint.edu/the-qanon-conspiracy-theory-a-security-threat-in-the-making/.

"Attila Hildmann in der Türkei: Haftbefehl nicht Vollstreckt." n.d. *Berlin.de.* Last Accessed June 14, 2022. https://www.berlin.de/aktuelles/berlin/kriminalitaet/6487076-4362932-attila-hildmann-in-der-tuerkei-haftbefeh.html.

Barkun, Michael. 2013. *A Culture of Conspiracy: Apocalyptic Visions in Contemporary America.* Vol. 15. California: University of California Press.

Benz, Wolfgang. 2021. *Querdenken: Protestbewegung zwischen Demokratieverachtung, Hass und Aufruhr.* Berlin: Metropol.

Birchall, Clare, and Peter Knight. 2022. "Do Your Own Research: Conspiracy Theories and the Internet." *Social Research: An International Quarterly* 89, no. 3: 579–605. doi:10.1353/sor.2022.0049.

Bothe, Detlef. 1991. "Neue Deutsche Heilkunde 1933–1945, dargestellt anhand der Zeitschrift 'Hippokrates' und der Entwicklung der volksheilkundlichen Laienbewegung." PhD diss., Freie Universität Berlin, published in *Abhand-*

*lungen zur Geschichte der Medizin und Naturwissenschaften 62*, Husum: Matthiesen Verlag.

Bratich, Jack Z. 2008. *Conspiracy Panics*. Albany: State University of New York Press.

Breuer, Stefan. 2005. "Von der antisemitischen zur völkischen Bewegung." *Aschkenas* 15, no. 2: 499–534.

Bricker, Brett, and Jacob Justice. 2019. "The Postmodern Medical Paradigm: A Case Study of Anti-MMR Vaccine Arguments." *Western Journal of Communication* 83, no. 2: 172–89.

Bruns, Axel, Stephen Harrington, and Edward Hurcombe. 2020. "'Corona? 5G? Or Both?': The Dynamics of COVID-19/5G Conspiracy Theories on Facebook." *Media International Australia* 177, no. 1: 12–29.

Butter, Michael. 2018. *'Nichts ist wie es scheint.' Über Verschwörungstheorien*. Berlin: Suhrkamp Verlag.

———. 2021. "Verschwörungstheorien: Eine Einführung." *Bundeszentrale für politische Bildung: Aus Politik und Zeitgeschichte*. August 27, 2021. https://www.bpb.de/shop/zeitschriften/apuz/verschwoerungstheorien-2021/339276/verschwoerungstheorien-eine-einfuehrung/.

Butter, Michael, and Peter Knight, eds. 2021. *Routledge Handbook of Conspiracy Theories*. London: Routledge.

———, eds. 2023. *Covid Conspiracy Theories in Global Perspective*. 1st ed. London: Routledge.

Cubitt, Geoffrey. 1989. "Conspiracy Myths and Conspiracy Theories." *Journal of the Anthropological Society of Oxford* 20, no. 1: 12–26.

Douglas, Karen M. 2021. "COVID-19 Conspiracy Theories." *Group Processes & Intergroup Relations* 24, no. 2: 270–5.

Douglas, Karen M., Robbie M. Sutton, and Aleksandra Cichocka. 2017. "The Psychology of Conspiracy Theories." *Current Directions in Psychological Science* 26, no. 6 (December): 538–42. https://doi.org/10.1177/0963721417718261.

Dredze, Mark, David A. Broniatowski, and Karen M. Hilyard. 2016. "Zika Vaccine Misconceptions: A Social Media Analysis." *Vaccine* 34, no. 30: 3441–2.

Dühring, Eugen. 1881. *Die Judenfrage als Racen-, Sitten- und Culturfrage: mit einer weltgeschichtlichen Antwort*. Karlsruhe: Reuther.

Durbach, Nadja. 2005. *Bodily Matters: The Anti-Vaccination Movement in England, 1853–1907*. Durham: Duke University Press.

Eckart, Wolfgang Uwe, and Robert Jütte. 2007. *Medizingeschichte–Eine Einführung*. Stuttgart: UTB-Verlag.

Ernst, Edward. 2001. "'Neue Deutsche Heilkunde': Complementary/ Alternative Medicine in the Third Reich." *Complementary Therapies in Medicine* 9, no. 1 (March): 49–51. https://doi.org/10.1054/ctim.2000.0416.

Flamm, Heinz, and Christian Vutuc. 2010. "Geschichte der Pocken-Bekämpfung in Österreich." *Wiener Klinische Wochenschrift* 122, no. 9 (May): 265–75.

Förster, Paul. 1900. *Pocken und Schutzimpfung.* Berlin: Deutschen Bundes der Impfgegner.

———. 1906. *Deutsche bildung, deutscher glaube, deutsche erziehung: eine streitschrift.* Leipzig: Wunderlich.

———. 1907. *Die Kunst des glücklichen Lebens. Mit einem Anhange: das Lachen; der Rausch, ein Evangelium für Enthaltsame; Autoritäten.* Berlin: Wilhelm Möller.

Frei, Nadine, and Oliver Nachtwey. 2022. "Quellen des 'Querdenkertums.' Eine politische Soziologie der Corona-Proteste in Baden-Württemberg." *SocArXiv Papers* (January). https://doi.org/10.31235/osf.io/8f4pb .

Frei, Nadine, Robert Schäfer, and Oliver Nachtwey. 2021. "Die Proteste gegen die Corona-Maßnahmen. Eine soziologische Annäherung." *Forschungsjournal Soziale Bewegungen* 34, no. 2: 249–58.

Hannig, Alma. 2020. "Antisemitismus und Populismus in Österreich: Zwei unzertrennliche Phänomene? – Eine geschichtswissenschaftliche Annäherung." In *Populismus—Kontroversen und Perspektiven: Ein wissenschaftliches Gesprächsangebot*, edited by Marina Fleck, Tobias Hirschmüller, and Thomas Hoffmann, 125–62. München: Akademische Verlagsgemeinschaft München.

Hildmann, Attila (@Attilahildmann). n.d. *Telegram Instant Messenger.* Last Accessed June 14, 2022. https://t.me/ATTILAHILDMANN.

Holzer, Boris. 2021. "Zwischen Protest und Parodie: Strukturen der 'Querdenken'-Kommunikation auf Telegram (und anderswo)." *Die Misstrauensgemeinschaft der Querdenker. Die Corona-Proteste aus kultur-und sozialwissenschaftlicher Perspektive:* 125–57.

Hotez, Peter J. 2020. "COVID19 Meets the Antivaccine Movement." *Microbes and Infection* 22, no. 4: 162.

Imhoff, Roland, and Martin Bruder. 2014. "Speaking (Un-)Truth to Power: Conspiracy Mentality as a Generalised Political Attitude." *European Journal of Personality* 28, no. 1 (January): 25–43.

Jolley, Daniel, and Karen M. Douglas. 2014. "The Effects of Anti-Vaccine Conspiracy Theories on Vaccination Intentions." *PLOS ONE* 9, no. 2 (February): e89177. https://doi.org/10.1371/journal.pone.0089177.

Kata, Anna. 2010. "A Postmodern Pandora's Box: Anti-Vaccination Misinformation on the Internet." *Vaccine* 28, no. 7: 1709–16.

———. 2012. "Anti-Vaccine Activists, Web 2.0, and the Postmodern Paradigm—An Overview of Tactics and Tropes Used Online by the Anti-Vaccination Movement." *Vaccine* 30, no. 25: 3778–89.

Keil, Jan-Gerrit. 2022. "Verschwörungserzählungen aus Sicht der Kriminalpsychologie und ihre besondere Rolle im Milieu von 'Reichsbürgern,' 'Impfgegnern' und 'QAnon-Anhängern.'" In *Schriften der Generalstaatsanwaltschaft Celle 6. Verschwörungstheorien: Ursprung—Anhänger—Bewältigung*, edited by Frank Lüttig and Jens Lehmann, 13–50. Baden-Baden: Nomos.

Kim, Louis, Shannon M. Fast, and Natasha Markuson. 2019. "Incorporating Media Data into a Model of Infectious Disease Transmission." *PLOS ONE* 14, no. 2 (February): e0197646. https://doi.org/10.1371/journal.pone.0197646.

Leask, Julie, and Simon Chapman. 2002. "'The Cold Hard Facts' Immunisation and Vaccine Preventable Diseases in Australia's Newsprint Media 1993–1998." *Social Science & Medicine* 54, no. 3: 445–57.

Lienert, Marina. 1998. "Das Rudolf-Heß-Krankenhaus in Dresden-Johannstadt—Zentrum der Neuen Deutschen Heilkunde im Dritten Reich." In *Dresden unterm Hakenkreuz*, edited by Reiner Pommerin, 209–26. Vienna: Böhlau Verlag.

Longerich, Peter. 2021. *Antisemitismus: eine deutsche Geschichte; von der Aufklärung bis Heute*. Munich: Siedler.

Miller, Joanne M., Kyle L. Saunders, and Christina E. Farhart. 2016. "Conspiracy Endorsement as Motivated Reasoning: The Moderating Roles of Political Knowledge and Trust." *American Journal of Political Science* 60, no. 4 (October): 824–44. https://doi.org/10.1111/ajps.12234.

Nan, Xiaoli, and Kelly Daily. 2015. "Biased Assimilation and Need for Closure: Examining the Effects of Mixed Blogs on Vaccine-Related Beliefs." *Journal of Health Communication* 20, no. 4: 462–71.

Nebe, Julia, Enno Schwanke, and Dominik Groß. 2021. "The Influence of Epidemics on the Concept of the Bogeyman: Images, Ideological Origins, and Interdependencies of the Anti-Vaccination Movement; The Example of the Political Agitator Paul Arthur Förster (1844–1925)." *Historical Social Research, Supplement* 33: 100–27. https://doi.org/10.12759/hsr.suppl.33.2021.100-127

Pfahl-Traughber, Armin. 1993. *Der antisemitisch-antifreimaurerische Verschwörungsmythos in der Weimarer Republik und im NS-Staat*. Vienna: Braunmüller.

———. 2015. "'Bausteine' zu einer Theorie über Verschwörungstheorien. Definitionen, Erscheinungsformen, Funktionen und Ursachen." In *Verschwörungstheorien. Theorie—Geschichte—Wirkung*, edited by Helmut Reinalter, 30–44. Innsbruck: Studienverlag.

Prooijen, Jan-Willem van, and Karen M. Douglas. 2017. "Conspiracy Theories as Part of History: The Role of Societal Crisis Situations." *Memory Studies* 10, no. 3 (July): 323–33. https://doi.org/10.1177/1750698017701615.

Pummerer, Lotte, Kevin Winter, and Kai Sassenberg. 2022. "Addressing Covid-19 Vaccination Conspiracy Theories and Vaccination Intentions." *European Journal of Health Communication* 3, no. 2: 1–12.

Pummerer, Lotte, Robert Böhm, Lau Lilleholt, Kevin Winter, Ingo Zettler, and Kai Sassenberg. 2020. "Conspiracy Theories and Their Societal Effects During the COVID-19 Pandemic." *PsyArXiv* (April). https://psyarxiv.com/y5grn/.

Puschner, Uwe, Walter Schmitz, and Justus H. Ulbricht. 2012. *Handbuch zur 'Völkischen Bewegung' 1871–1918*. Berlin: K. G. Saur.

Rensmann, Lars. 2008. "'Globalisierung' und Antisemitismus in rechtsextremen Parteien." In *Feindbild Judentum: Antisemitismus in Europa*, edited by Lars Rensmann and Julius Schoeps, 399–453. Berlin: VBB.

Rutter, Martin. 2020. " Freunderl, Globalisten und 'Corona Diktatoren' unter sich." *Direkt Demokratisch*. April 7, 2020, 01:02 a.m. Telegram, https://t.me/MartinRutter/55.

———. n.d. "Telegramm-Gruppen." *Direkt Demokratisch*. Last Accessed June 14, 2022. https://www.direktdemokratisch.jetzt/telegram-gruppen/.

Safford, Thomas G., Lawrence C. Hamilton, and Emily H. Whitmore. 2017. "The Zika Virus Threat: How Concerns about Scientists May Undermine Efforts to Combat the Pandemic." *Carsey Research: Regional Issue Brief* 49 (Spring). https://dx.doi.org/10.34051/p/2020.288.

Salzborn, Samuel. 2021. "Verschwörungsmythen und Antisemitismus." *Aus Politik und Zeitgeschichte* 35, no. 36: 41–7.

Schwab, Klaus, and Thierry Malleret. 2020. *Covid-19: The Great Reset*. Geneva: World Economic Forum.

Shahsavari, Shadi, Pavan Holur, Tianyi Wang, Timothy R. Tangherlini, and Vwani Roychowdhury. 2020. "Conspiracy in the Time of Corona: Automatic Detection of Emerging COVID-19 Conspiracy Theories in Social Media and the News." *Journal of Computational Social Science* 3, no. 2: 279–317.

Sharma, Megha, Kapil Yadav, Nitika Yadav, and Keith C. Ferdinand. 2017. "Zika Virus Pandemic—Analysis of Facebook as a Social Media Health Information Platform." *American Journal of Infection Control* 45, no. 3 (March): 301–2.

Simonsen, Kjetil Braut. 2020. "Antisemitism and Conspiracism." In *Routledge Handbook of Conspiracy Theories*, edited by Michael Butter and Peter Knight, 1st ed., 357–70. London: Routledge.

Smallpage, Steven M., Adam M. Enders, and Joseph E. Uscinski. 2017. "The Partisan Contours of Conspiracy Theory Beliefs." *Research & Politics* 4, no. 4 (December): 1–7. https://doi.org/10.1177/2053168017746554.

Smith, Naomi, and Tim Graham. 2019. "Mapping the Anti-Vaccination Movement on Facebook." *Information, Communication & Society* 22, no. 9: 1310–27.

Sutton, Robbie M., and Karen M. Douglas. 2020. "Conspiracy Theories and the Conspiracy Mindset: Implications for Political Ideology." *Current Opinion in Behavioral Sciences* 34 (February): 118–22. https://doi.org/10.1016/j.cobeha.2 020.02.015.

Thießen, Malte. 2017. *Immunisierte Gesellschaft: Impfen in Deutschland im 19. und 20. Jahrhundert*. Vol. 225. Göttingen: Vandenhoeck & Ruprecht.

———. 2021. *Auf Abstand: eine Gesellschaftsgeschichte der Coronapandemie*. Frankfurt: Campus Verlag.

Trobisch, Andreas, Daniela Sabine Klobassa, H. Gschiel, M. Wassermann-Neuhold, and W. Zenz. 2019. "Analyse des Masernausbruches 2015 in der Steiermark." *Monatsschrift Kinderheilkunde* 167, no. 40 (January): 46–50. htt ps://doi.org/10.1007/s00112-017-0340-y .

Tschiggerl, Martin. 2023. "Bill Gates, Impfungen und die New World Order. Verschwörungstheorien zu COVID-19 in Sozialen Medien." In *Superspreader: Popkultur und mediale Öffentlichkeiten im Angesicht der Pandemie*, edited by Tobias Eichinger, Arno Görgen, and Eugen Pfister. Bielefeld: transcript.

Ullah, Irfan, K. S. Khan, M. J. Tahir, A. Ahmed, and H. Harapan. 2021. "Myths and Conspiracy Theories on Vaccines and COVID-19: Potential Effect on Global Vaccine Refusals." *Vacunas* 22, no. 2: 93–7.

Uscinski, Joseph E., Adam M. Enders, Casey Klofstad, Michelle Seelig, John Funchion, Caleb Everett, Stefan Wuchty, Kamal Premaratne, and Manohar Murthi. 2020. "Why Do People Believe COVID-19 Conspiracy Theories?" *Harvard Kennedy School Misinformation Review* 1, no. 3 (April). https://misinforeview.hks.harvard.edu/article/why-do-people-believe-covid-19-conspiracy-theories/.

Van Prooijen, Jan-Willem. 2019. "Belief in Conspiracy Theories: Gullibility or Rational Skepticism?" In *The Social Psychology of Gullibility: Conspiracy The-*

ories, *Fake News and Irrational Beliefs*, edited by Joseph P. Forgas and Roy Baumeister, 319–32. New York: Routledge.

Wetzel, Juliane. 2021. "Bindekitt für Verdrossene und Verweigerer." In *Querdenken: Protestbewegung zwischen Demokratieverachtung, Hass und Aufruhr*, edited by Wolfgang Benz, 55–75. Berlin: Metropol.

Wolff, Eberhard. 1996. "Medizinkritik der Impfgegner im Spannungsfeld zwischen Lebenswelt und Wissenschaftsorientierung." In *Medizinkritische Bewegungen im Deutschen Reich (ca. 1870 – ca. 1933)*, edited by Martin Dinges, 79–126. Stuttgart: Franz Steiner Verlag.

"www.impfopfer.info. WIR Gemeinsam für die FREIHEIT." n.d. *Telegram Instant Messenger*. Last Accessed June 14, 2022. https://t.me/Impfschaden_D _AUT_CH.

# 7. The Quest for Tropical Nature: Utopia and Socio-Spatial Dynamics in Brazil during the COVID-19 Pandemic

*Danielle Heberle Viegas*

Mobility did not seem to be a top-of-mind concern among the many brought forth by the COVID-19 pandemic. Expressions such as 'quarantine,' 'home office,' 'lockdown' and others that became part of the pandemic lexicon seem to be more essential in any draft version of a social analysis of the pandemic than any mention of population movements. However, as with most generalizations, this is partially a red herring: in a report published in 2020, the International Organization for Migration (IOM) highlighted that, while global mobility declined, the catastrophic effects of the pandemic on migrants have never been more severe, revealing the importance of making a more comprehensive analysis of these mobilities (Benton et al. 2020). The situation in Latin America has been described as "mobility to immobility"[1] by multiple sources who reported on and denounced the drama faced by those trapped in refuge or displacement when countries suddenly closed their borders.

In addition to immigration in the strictest sense of the word, other phenomena broadly related to population mobility have also been observed since the beginning of the pandemic. These have ranged from new configurations of commuting patterns in metropolitan regions, returning migrations—i.e., people leaving cities towards the countryside, counteracting trends seen throughout the twentieth century—through to occasional shifts to areas away from large urban centers. When reporting on these, the media wasted no time splashing the supposed 'new phenomena' across the frontpages of their newspapers, websites, and social media profiles: In Spain, *El País* described

---

1    For more information, see Álvarez Velasco, Soledad. 2020. "COVID-19 and (Im)mobility in the Americas."

the return to the countryside as a modern utopia (De Llano 2021), while Germany's famous news magazine *Der Spiegel* and the UK's BBC emphasized how properties in the outskirts of metropolises have seen skyrocketing prices amid stronger demand for living in green areas (Jauernig 2021; Brennan 2020).

In Brazil, regularly reported as one of the countries most affected by COVID-19 due to the number of deaths it caused, stories on changes in population movements were highlighted by national media from the very first months of the pandemic: On June 26, 2020, the frontpage of the Brazilian newspaper *Zero Hora* detailed government concerns regarding population movement from state capitals towards the Atlantic coast. Another one, *O Estado de São Paulo*, featured a story on the "New Rural" phenomenon and its apparent rise during the pandemic. As a whole, these reports were basically clues pointing to a larger shift: increased mobility towards places generically associated with idealized expressions of nature outside the country's major cities. The finding is supported by figures provided by observatories, tourist agencies, real estate companies and academic research (Nicolelis et al. 2021). The drivers of these movements fall into a wide range of categories, including tourism and its multiple variations, rentals offered by global platforms, and increased purchases of homes in gated communities. Although this cannot yet be statistically determined, such populational flows are a key factor in understanding a trend that has roots in the past and portrays the present of Brazilian society and the country's relationship with tropical nature.

Many small- and mid-sized cities or more distant regions have become compelling options for people wary of the risks posed by most major Brazilian urban centers. Violence, unemployment, high costs of living and the pandemic have coalesced into a perfect storm of legitimate reasons for escaping the urban. Moreover, lower-density urban agglomerations and rural areas have come to be seen as havens where norms concerning social isolation are seen as more lax, making for visions—albeit mostly unspoken—of utopian cultures bringing a novel, healthier ambience for those looking for a countervailing portrait to the current social and health crises.

In light of the above, I sought to investigate at least two major trends that emerged during the pandemic and that seem to signal this shift: increased nature tourism and expanded acquisitions of subdivisions in gated communities usually called *condomínios fechados* ('closed condominiums') in the countryside. Both can be understood as hygienist patterns entangled with the history of biopolitics in Brazil, revealing long-standing processes of othering. They are based on social and natural segregation in which eco-friendly neoliberal subjectivities and greenwashing are bound to the imagination of a healthy and controlled nature, and spatial militarization emerges in regard to rural idyllic areas.

This chapter is based on interviews conducted with representatives from the real estate and tourism sectors in Brazil, compiling a total of eleven testimonies by technicians and specialists from the following institutions and entities: Associação Brasileira de Incorporadoras Imobiliárias (Brazilian Association of Real Estate Developers), Associação de Empresas de Loteamento e Desenvolvimento Urbano do Brasil (Brazilian Association of Subdivision and Urban Development Companies [Aelo]), Instituto Brasil Rural (The Rural Brazil Institute), Confederação Nacional dos Municípios (National Confederation of Municipalities), Associação Brasileira de Turismo de Aventura (Brazilian Ecotourism and Adventure Tourism Trade Association [ABETA]), Associação Brasileira das Operadoras de Turismo (Brazilian Association of Tour Operators), Ministério do Turismo (Ministry of Tourism), Rede Brasileira de Trilhas (Brazilian Trails Network), Instituto Copenhagen (Copenhagen Institute), and Brain: Inteligência Estratégica (Brain Institute: Strategic Intelligence).[2] In addition, I also conducted desk research on three of Brazil's major newspapers (*Estado de S. Paulo*, *Folha de São Paulo* and *O Globo*) for the words 'refuge,' 'nature' and 'pandemic' (and related terms).

To understand the mobilities of COVID-19, one must first formulate a critique of the discourses on nature, the tropical and its propagation to landscapes and times, done here chiefly through the idea of translocality (Freitag and von Oppen 2010). The concept seeks to explain the tension between movement and order and is particularly sensitive to the attempt of making sense of a world full of fluxes—something especially important as the pandemic reinforced the notion of control over spaces and bodies, of where, when and how to go (and, above all, where, when and how *not* to go). In addition, the paper draws on theoretical approaches of environmental history as well as urban studies. Since the 1990s, a line of thought has emerged that looks at the concept of nature from a cultural standpoint, providing an interesting counternarrative to the usual nature *versus* culture binary and marking the beginning of environmental history as an independent area of study. This "cultural turn" has argued that nature is a social construct, not a given entity explainable *per se* (Carey 2009).

---

2    My translation.

It is worth asking, therefore: What can historians tell us about this populational drive towards nature? What does this mean for the "euphoria of movement, mobility and circulation" that is a historical mainstay of the global community (Conrad 2016)? In an attempt to address these issues, this chapter describes the phenomenon of nature-induced mobility during the COVID-19 pandemic in Brazil first in general terms, followed by a more detailed presentation of two selected case studies. My aim is to understand which social meanings of tropical nature and utopia have been mobilized to generate this drive, as well as to describe how those contemporary experiences have been heavily informed by lifestyle aspirations (Vieira 2018).

To achieve these ends, I have structured this chapter as follows: After an initial section contextualizing Brazil's internal association of (tropical) nature and utopia and the role of the coast in this social construct, I present the first illustrative example, namely nature tourism, and proceed to discuss how the pandemic has reinforced the idyllic ideal of the beach as a place of redemption from the urban problems of Brazil (Corbin 1988). In the third section, I postulate how the notion of tropical nature has evolved in the expansion of gated communities in Brazil that tout the so-called invented environment. Finally, I compare both case studies to conclude with a discussion of how different utopian cultures can help explain these mobilities, driven by the desire to find an imagined type of safe nature in Brazil, and how both cases help put class segregation in relief as this reimagining of the colonial past collides with green capitalism and neoliberal environmentalism (Acker, Kaltmeier, and Tittor 2016).

## A Few Remarks on Utopia and Tropical Nature in Brazil

South America has historically been an important stage for utopian experiences: From the Guarani native 'land without pain' to the Jesuit missions, utopia has remained a central historical tenet of the continent. The invention of America was accompanied by the unleashing of European imaginative potentials, followed by many tragic events. Nature has been a cornerstone of the mythical makeup of utopia across America, from the cities beyond the mountain and the conquest of the West in the US to the legends of the 'Eldorado' in the Amazon.

Brazil's very name is an allusion to a tree (*Paubrasilia echinatta*), and it is a point of agreement among researchers that every image forged in our heads about the daily life of Brazilian colonial society has, in its most subtle substrate, several material elements whose archeology takes us to an inexorable starting point: the tree (Cabral 2014, 59). The formation of the State and the negotiation of a national identity was always mediated by reflections on nature and its role—sometimes as a driver of development, sometimes as a reason for its failure. Nature has generally been seen as a mythical constituent of Brazilian national identity and it has historically been considered a setting for the realization of utopias (Murari 2009), even if this imagery of the purity of nature was partially mutated at times—during the developmentalist project, for example. Many authors have been looking at these utopias as a transnational phenomenon connecting Brazil, Africa and Lusophone African countries (Bethencourt 2015).

This view of nature as redemption and the quest for so-called natural places has not been circumscribed to Brazil, of course. From the American West to the bucolic old England of green and the *Deutscher Wald* (The German Forest), an intricate web connects our collective memory with the environment. What sets Brazilian identity apart from those is that it is not associated with a general idea of nature, but rather with the idea of *tropical* nature, the main 'regionalizing' element of the theme. This is well rooted in the country's history, spanning from the deliberate creation of demographic voids to advance internal colonialism and land occupancy public policies during the XXth century, to the aristocratic tradition of building summer palaces and the massive exploitation of Brazilian natural resources in the 1890s, all driven by the imagined notion that the country's interior could hold an infinite variety of landscapes and societies.

In fact, there is significant literature in Brazilian social thought wherein the country is stereotypically described as a promising, harmonious and healthy land due to its unique natural traits. Varnhagen rejected the impossibility of tropical civilization, but found it difficult to achieve (1870); Gilberto Freyre proposed a "racial democracy" built on the idea of Lusotropicalism and the presumed success of Portuguese imperialism in controlling tropical geographies (2011); Oswald de Andrade (2009) used tropical nature as a motivation to envisage syncretic political futures based on the modern world and indigenous thought. Lastly, Stefan Zweig (2013) presents a foreigner's view, praising Brazil's luxurious, "emotional," "sensual" tropical nature as a contrast to modern European rationalism and bureaucratism. In the twentieth century, cultural movements such as Tropicália and the boom in international tourism compounded the discourses and practices that for centuries centralized tropicality as an essentially Brazilian landmark. As can be seen, the image of a tropical country deeply rooted in the nation's utopian ethos has been constantly mobilized.

The coast plays a very particular role in this narrative, and its connection with the notion of paradise completely eradicated the idea of beaches as threatening places (Kaenzig and Piguet 2011). Instead, imagery of the coast as a place of redemption and health has been explored to the fullest. The origins of this movement in the country date back to the late nineteenth century, when Brazil's first seaside resorts were opened on the Atlantic coast and vacationing there was lauded for its therapeutic purposes (often prescribed by doctors at the time). The marketing of these seaside resorts often projected a social space free from urban problems, a small-scale, short-lived utopia lasting for a summer (Schossler 2021). These images are still widely represented in contemporary experiences in Brazil, whether for the promotion of nature tourism or the so-called green capitalism, touting urban ecosystems in gated communities (as exemplified in the case studies that follow).

## "I Live in a Tropical Country"[3]: The *Corona Paradise* Project

One of the most remarkable campaigns promoting nature-induced mobility and tourism in Brazil during the COVID-19 pandemic was the one launched by the brewery *Modelo*. The company, originally founded in Mexico in the 1920s, developed a marketing project ironically called *Corona Paradise*[4] to promote one of its top-selling beers worldwide: *Corona*. On its website, the project is advertised as a selection of curated destinations "for those looking for an authentic connection with nature in settings that are true paradises in Brazil" (Corona Paradise 2020, my translation).[5] Launched in mid-2020, the platform has since grown and lists a number of locations. It self-describes as a "website partly focused on travel and experiences" where "users can find offers of various stay options, such as houses, hotels, guest houses and hostels; and experiences, such

---

3    The title is part of the lyrics to the song *País Tropical*, composed by famous Brazilian singer Jorge Ben.

4    See: "Corona Paradise" from *The Summer Hunter* (2023).

5    This and all the following quotes from the original website were translated from the original Portuguese by the author. Please see: "Corona Paradise" from *The Summer Hunter* (2023).

as tours, classes, workshops and much more" (Corona Paradise 2020, my translation). Two things immediately stand out here: the launch of a project to promote travel and accommodation at the height of the pandemic in Brazil, and the promise of an authentic connection with nature.

The destinations listed on the platform are divided into five categories: adventure tourism/ecotourism, nature/disconnect, sport in nature, wellness, and fun. The selection does not include destinations located close to the Amazon rainforest, the Pampa, or the Brazilian rural world. *Corona Paradise*'s concept of nature tourism relies on destinations in a single setting: beaches, bringing a modern patina to the notion of the ocean as a problem-free space that emerged in the last decades of the nineteenth century.

The website's vocabulary is steeped in tropicality, often relying on racist and colonial tropes of the 'paradise lost' of Brazil's pristine coast (and forests), ignoring the political and ontological existence of indigenous cultures and natures (Cronon 1996, 7). The role of coloniality or colonial legacies in producing racialized social classifications and spatial inequalities is clear, for instance, when the website describes the island of Boipeba, in Bahia, as follows: "the feeling is that little has changed since Velha Boipeba[6] was founded by the Portuguese in 1537" (Corona Paradise 2020, my translation). Referring to Pipa, a beach on the coast of the northeastern state of Rio Grande do Norte, the website once again sings the praises of European presence:

> While nowadays it is normal everywhere to be served by a guy with an Italian accent in any corner of the northeastern coast, it was at Pipa that the invasion of the 'sweet barbarians' first made its mark. With its breathtaking sequence of bays and cliffs less than two hours from Natal's international airport, this *Potiguar*[7] beach was popular with Europeans, who helped internationalize the local cuisine while the village has developed (almost) without losing its essence. (Corona Paradise 2020, my translation)

The search for the tropical must be seen above all as socially constructed and the apparent naturalization is the result of long-standing colonial discourses (Ross 2017). The idea of the tropical purely natural environment is embedded in the production of tropicality (McNeill and Mauldin 2012), a concept scholars have recently developed to criticize discourses, practices, and images of the

---

6    'Old Boipeba.'
7    Indigenous word for natives of Rio Grande do Norte.

tropics based on colonialist and ethnocentric tropes (Monzote 2018). The tropics have been objectified as an ambiguous geography whose main features involve luxurious and natural landscapes. During the time of the COVID-19 pandemic, tropical imagery strengthened this colonial view, intensifying the existing disparities in socio-ecological relationships by presenting an exclusive and alluring landscape as its premise. The mobility dynamics that emerged were marked by many bodies being in denial of other bodies and they exacerbated processes of social exclusion by means of private militarization and greenwashing.

Lockdown experiences in Brazil were framed as voluntary acts, experienced as such by economically well-off groups who had more than one residence and sufficient home-office space. The *Corona Paradise* project often describes idyllic well-being and relaxation while connecting work-related terms to the touristic experience, touting expressions such as "resort office" and "workcation," among others. In addition, portrayals of the daily lives of professionals and influencers who have chosen remote work have been published. The website aligns with a broader trend for increased nature tourism in Brazil, as highlighted by Vinícius Viegas, the current President of the Brazilian Ecotourism and Adventure Tourism Trade Association (ABETA):

> So, what I've realized is that tourism is a luxury item. Traveling is a luxury item. During the pandemic, there were certain things that people couldn't do and that made traveling, the fact of being in another destination, a little more of a sophisticated luxury, let's say, something more elitist. And the artists, the influencers, they couldn't leave Brazil, they couldn't travel the world like they used to. So what we saw was a massive promotion of places like Lençóis Maranhenses in the state of Maranhão, and Jalapão, along the coast of the state of Alagoas. We saw many artists and famous people going to these places. And that ultimately helped intensify visits to certain places, you know? Traveling turned out to be much more of a luxury item, with a lot more value than it had had before. (Vinícius Viegas 2021, my translation)[8]

---

8    "Então, o que eu percebo é que o turismo é um artigo de luxo. Viajar é um artigo de luxo. Durante a pandemia, as pessoas não puderam fazer algumas coisas e isso fez com que o fato de viajar, o fato de estar em outro destino, é, se tornasse um luxo um pouco mais sofisticado, vamos dizer assim, um luxo mais elitizado. E os artistas, influenciadores, eles não puderam ir pra fora do Brasil, eles não puderam rodar o mundo, como eles estão acostumados. e o que a gente viu foi a promoção massiva de Lençóis Maranhenses, litoral de Alagoas, Jalapão, então a gente viu muitos artistas, muita gente famosa indo pra esses lugares. E isso acabou, é, ajudando a intensificar a visitação em

Nature tourism and its multiple variables were put in sharp relief as tourism faced a worldwide crisis, having become one of the main alternatives for the recovery of the sector in Brazil. Specialists report that the search for nature tourism has suddenly increased due to the allure of outdoor activities, travel in small groups, accommodation in family guest houses and the general possibility of enjoying the outdoors after several months of unofficial lockdowns.

Marina Figueiredo, Vice-President of the Brazilian Association of Tour Operators and member of the movement *Supera Turismo Brasil* ("Recovering Tourism in Brazil"), explained:

> Nature destinations, at first, were also destinations that were the most sought after, and have continued to be so until today. It's like a big trend: people still want places close to nature, open places, that bring a greater sense of security, you know? Being in an environment that is more open... Smaller places. So, at first, that was it. And, obviously, as things went on and evolved, new things started to open up, things started to grow again. But it's important that we realize that, even today, with people returning to making those longer trips and so on, the experience they had of that little place near their home will not be forgotten. (2021, my translation)[9]

But while the beach continues to be perceived as this ideal tropical paradise—as the *Corona Paradise* project reaffirmed—it has now begun to face competition: new areas that seek to combine Brazilians' preference for the coast with a much-desired sense of security and exclusivity, giving new meanings to historical social practices related to tropical nature in the country.

---

alguns locais, sabe? Então, viajar acabou se tornando um artigo de luxo muito mais, é, com muito mais valor do que era antes, sabe?" (Vinícius Viegas 2021).

9    "Destinos de natureza, também, num primeiro momento, foram destinos, ahn, mais buscados. Eles continuam hoje, é, como uma grande tendência; as pessoas continuam ainda querendo locais próximos à natureza, locais abertos, que dá essa sensação maior de segurança, né? Estar num ambiente, é, mais aberto, locais menores. Então, num primeiro momento, foi isso. E, obviamente, conforme as coisas foram, é, evoluindo, né, e foram tendo novas aberturas, isso volta a crescer, mas é importante que a gente percebe que, mesmo hoje, as pessoas voltando a fazer essas viagens mais longas e tudo mais, o conhecimento que elas tiveram daquele lugarzinho ali do lado da casa delas, não vai ser esquecido" (Marina Figueiredo 2021).

## *Fugere Urbem*: Gated Communities and Dreams of Mobility and Security in Brazil

Like many gated communities in inner São Paulo State, *Fazenda da Grama* is clearly aimed at high-income future residents. Unlike others of its kind, however, it offers something rather special: an exclusive artificial beach with waves and native Atlantic forest vegetation. Built in Itupeva—a city seventy-three kilometers from the state capital—the unique gated community was created in 2019. When the pandemic hit Brazil by February 2020, the cost per square meter for a piece of land in Fazenda da Grama was R$ 300, with the smallest lots measuring 2,200 square meters (approximately 23,600 sqft). A week later, that same per-square-meter price went up to around R$ 1,000, or about R$ 2 million just to acquire the bare land at the minimum size offered.

Among its amenities, *Fazenda da Grama* features a huge artificial lake with "a thousand waves per hour with quality similar to that of the ocean."[10] According to the website, the gated community is "the only condominium in the world with beach, golf and horseback riding facilities." Some inconveniences of tropical climate were addressed by technology: the sand, for example, does not get hot; the size of the waves can be adjusted in advance; and the promotional photos do not show any people at the beach—a clear attempt to differentiate the exclusive project from public beaches, usually crowded in Brazil.

The artificial waves and temperature-controlled sand offer a stark example of the concept of 'invented natures,' currently at the forefront of discourses on urban planning, development and smart cities. *Fazenda da Gama*'s offers share similarities with those of many other residential developments worldwide that advertise greenhouses, swimming pools and amusement parks all conceived to recreate climatic environments not found locally. The gated community also offers a private forest constituting an object of "nature-spatial civilization" as described by Olaf Kaltmeier (2021): "in the sense of hygienic improvement and economic utilization promoted by a targeted biopolitics of orderly foresting." As its website announces: "Through forest trails, residents can connect with nature and will be able to go on walks and plant and harvest their own food, learning how it is produced."

In addition to the green marketing promises, *Fazenda da Grama*'s advertising materials also add an element of class differentiation by emphasizing its

---

10    This and all the following quotes from the website were translated from the original Portuguese by the author.

investment in safety. The social strata most attracted to these mobilities have been the rich, as can be seen in the price of the properties and plots of land and the high-level amenities. Places such as *Fazenda da Gama* illustrate both the recent trend for the construction of 'artificial' environments and the importance of the notion of social segregation (as exemplified by the emphasis on the gated community aspect). The prices and the very architectural makeup of the model units are clearly targeted at upper-class future inhabitants. People attracted to these developments have in common the desire to seek out alternatives to the big city lifestyles which also serve as a symbol of their socioeconomic wealth; they wish to both show off their economic power and claim they are contributing to global environmental causes—all while enjoying the latest technological comforts (i.e., isolated, but still fully connected).

The civil construction sector ended 2020 with profits up ten percent, buoyed by real estate sales at an all-time-high even amid one of the biggest economic and health crises in contemporary Brazilian history. Although sales were up across several segments, the product that topped them all were plots of land in gated communities. Caio Portugal, president of the Brazilian Association of Subdivision and Urban Development Companies (Aelo), explains:

> Looking at it from the perspective of receptivity, the product that has been most consumed would be plots of land inside gated communities. Subdivisions inside gated communities. We saw the phenomenon of [developments] running out of stock. Whoever had this product—like, within, I don't know, a forty or fifty kilometer range from large cities, or even within these large cities—they practically ran out of stock. So now we are seeing this phenomenon, that is the high number of houses being built in these places, either by investors who realized that this was what consumers were looking for, or end consumers who saw that they could move out. (Caio Portugal 2021, my translation)[11]

---

11    "Se a gente pegar do ponto de vista de absorção, o produto que foi mais consumido foi o loteamento de acesso controlado, né. *O loteamento fechado de condomínios, que a gente viu não só o fenômeno de zerar os estoques, então, quem tinha este produto numa—a gente, há um eixo aí de, sei lá, 40, 50km de grandes cidades, ou mesmo dentro dessas grandes cidades—, teve praticamente uma zeragem desse estoque, né? E a gente vê agora o fenômeno que é o volume de casas sendo construídas nesses locais, sejam por investidores que perceberam que o público consumidor está buscando isso, seja o próprio consumidor final, que viu que podia mudar, né?" (Caio Portugal 2021).

Relying on statistics from far-reaching surveys prepared by his company (which has applied over 30,000 questionnaires and conducted in-depth interviews), Marcos Kathalian, a partner at Brain (a company that maps trends on the Brazilian real estate market), states that the expansion of the market was driven by three factors: two economic ones and one behavioral in nature. The financial factors were the low interest rates for acquiring property and high capital liquidity in middle- and upper-class households in Brazil. The political environment also played a role: Restrictions on foreign travel as well as certain contraints within Brazil itself were also conditioning elements. But there was also a third factor, the one of most interest to historians as it reveals the historical meanings and connections of these movements. There was an important behavioral component to this expansion, driven by the profound isolation experienced by the population that was stuck at home during the pandemic. In Kathalian words: "there was an intense search for horizontality, to leave the apartments of the big cities, to move into a house, to more spacious environments, environments with more green, more light; a sort of yearning to find space, a desire to find green" (Marcos Kathalian 2021, my translation).[12]

Gated communities reproduce colonial politics of exclusion and racialization by granting this private space to some, while denying it to many others, whose bodies are also persecuted and expelled in public spaces through gentrification and beach privatization policies. This process is entangled with necropolitics, a term developed by Achille Mbembe (2016) which considers the relationship between politics, the body, and death on the periphery of modernity/coloniality. It is a very pertinent concept to explore the Brazilian situation (not only, but especially) during the pandemic of COVID-19. Worldwide, the country was notoriously renowned for practices classified as necropolitical, including the public downplay of vaccine effects by the Brazilian president, Jair Messias Bolsonaro. Necropolitics is entangled in the creation of spaces of difference and exclusion. According to Mbembe, "the ultimate expression of power is the ability to dictate who may live and who must die .... To exercise sovereignty is to exercise control over mortality and to define life as the deployment and manifestation of power" (2016, 123, my translation).

---

12    "Houve aí uma procura intensa por horizontalidade, por sair de apartamentos nas grandes cidades, ir para casas, ambientes mais espaçosos, ambientes com mais verde, com mais iluminação, numa espécie de angústia de espaço e angústia de verde" (Marcos Kathalian 2021).

The financing of the territories for gated communities perpetuates the production of racialized identities, keeping in operation the racial genocide that is at the base of the country's formation since the beginning of the colonization process. However, gated communities cannot be understood as a producer of racialization, but rather as an actualizer, through these ever-repeated practices of exclusion and control. This process contributes to a heterogeneity of techniques to produce the social and ontological hierarchization of individuals, including their location, function, and access to city spaces.

The notion of cities as propagators of diseases and—by contrast—of the countryside and green spaces as places of redemption is nothing new, neither in Brazil nor worldwide. Brazil has seen the creation of luxury gated communities in green environments for the last three decades. The peculiarity of these condominiums in Brazil is that, in addition to (and despite) their access to green areas, they also bear stark signs of urban militarization: cameras and security guards are ubiquitous, with stringent alarms and strict digital controls for entry and exit (Graham 2016). Such devices are part of an architecture that serves to separate the bodies that deserve to live from the useless bodies: from naked life or, as Butler (2016) says, from "precarious life." Security mechanisms, including surveillance and other control mechanisms that often become mechanisms for abuse of power (Ritter 2014), are justified as forms of protection of those who deserve to live, while spaces like bike paths, outdoor gyms, lawns and parks are constructed to allow them to enhance their living conditions further.

These gated communities show that it is not sufficient for these groups to just visit nature (a role that could be played by public parks in the capitals, for example). It is imperative for upper-class citizens to own these plots of land, which must come with the assurance of safety that clearly indicates the social class of the people making use of that nature. Pedro Menezes, Director of *Rede Trilhas* (the Trails Network), adds an important reminder: "In Brazil, most protected areas are located in urban centers. Therefore, there would be no drive to leave cities if the purpose was merely to find more green" (2021, my translation).[13] Gated communities, utopian pasts, greenwashing, and urban policies are perhaps creating the conditions for a nature in which enjoyment of natural/invented sustainable environments, ecological practices and eco-friendly

---

13   "No Brasil, a maioria das áreas protegidas está localizada em centros urbanos. Portanto, não haveria motivo para deixar as cidades se o objetivo fosse apenas encontrar mais verde" (Pedro Menezes 2021).

subjectivities walk hand-in-hand with spatial militarization and social exclusion.

## Conclusion

Prestigious Brazilian journalist Marco de Sá Corrêa once wrote that "when I was a child, the forest was for the poor; today, the forest is for the rich."[14] The statement—coincidentally directly quoted by one of the interviewees—speaks to at least three important elements of the displacements discussed in this chapter: Firstly, the recurrent idea that nature lies beyond the city and must be sought after and/or tamed; secondly, the social uses of nature: what and who it serves; and finally, 'which' nature is being talked about.

The search for natural spaces is a trend seen far beyond the borders of Brazil; valuing nature as an integral part of national identity and culture is a global phenomenon; the causal relationship between displacements and natural spatialities that Brazil sees is by no means a localized, one-of-a-kind development. That said, even if these arguments for a global point of view on this topic are valid, they cannot fully explain all the national and regional issues involved. While the search for natural spaces—and particularly for natural spaces outside metropolitan regions—has not been specific to Brazil, the debate took on some very interesting contours; the result of a combination of the worldwide fame of Brazili's tropical nature, the dire scenario the country faced with the COVID-19 pandemic, and the various projects of its past that sought to correlate nature with utopia. But what exactly connects biopolitics, mobility, nature and the pandemic in Brazil?

The peculiarities I highlighted sought chiefly to ensure the discussion of the social uses of nature in Brazil (past and present) and the strong influence of colonialism on the notion of tropicality in the country. Biopolitics is exercised, in the Brazilian context, inseparably from the colonial matrix, which produces racialized and classified identities in order to hierarchize existences and to determine which bodies remain outside the limits of what is understood as a healthy territory, free of dangers and guided by well-being.

By seeing displacements merely as a result of chance, or just the drive of socially privileged sectors of society to seek more comfortable living elsewhere, one runs the risk of arriving at generalizations that are only partially

---

14    This and all other non-English citations hereafter have been translated by the author.

true. Avoiding that, in the case of Brazil, means attempting to understand the different meanings of nature in a country deeply associated with tropicalism, and why nature is associated with well-being. The latter view, for example, is certainly not an absolute paradigm for social groups other than the middle-classes; those who make their living off the land or even have a holistic world-view of nature, such as indigenous peoples, see nature as much more than a space to be used.

To understand the so-called *green grabbing* process, one must "attend to both the nature of new political economies and discourses around nature, and how they play into regionally or locally specific histories of environments, land use, governance and agrarian relations" (Fairbairn et al. 2014). The environment started to figure prominently in the agenda of movements, practices, and groups beginning in the 1970s, subsequently becoming a full-fledged political discourse and influencing everything from marketing strategies to tourism practices (especially, but not exclusively, ecological and environmental tourism), "responding to a process of adjustment of the market itself to the new environmental imperatives" (Howlett and Raglon 1992).

Such movements may be explained by the expansion of the Global North's "imperial way of living," leading elites to seek to live in more affluent southern countries (Brand and Wissen 2021). As such, these "dreams of connectivity" and enjoyment of nature, as mentioned by Farish Noor (2020), clearly happen against a backdrop of social differentiation, reinforcing discourses of neoliberal environmentalism in which sustainability is traded as a commodity, with the social justice dimension thereof often left unaddressed. These ideas about tropical nature have played a central role in the development of Brazilian cities and their surrounding regions during the pandemic, shedding light on an issue of major interest for urban and environmental historians seeking to research the past, present and future of utopian ideals and the global connections between them.

## Works Cited

Acker, Antoine, Olaf Kaltmeier, and Anne Tittor. 2016. "The Social Production of Nature Between Coloniality and Capitalism (Introduction)." *Forum for InterAmerican Research* 9, no. 2: 5–24. http://interamerica.de/volume-9-2/9-2 contents/.

Álvarez Velasco, Soledad. 2020. "COVID-19 and (Im)mobility in the Americas." *(Im)mobility in the Americas*. 2020. https://www.inmovilidadamericas.org/?lang=en.

Benton, Meghan, Jeanne Batalova, Samuel Davidoff-Gore, and Timo Schmidt. 2020. *COVID-19 and the State of Global Mobility in 2020*. IOM Publications Platform, https://publications.iom.int/books/COVID-19-and-state-global-mobility-2020.

Bethencourt, Francisco. 2015. *Utopia in Portugal, Brazil and Lusophone African Countries*. Oxford: Lang.

Brand, Ulrich, and Markus Wissen. 2021. *The Imperial Mode of Living: Everyday Life and the Ecological Crisis of Capitalism*. Edited by Barbara Jungwirth, translated by Zachary Murphy King. London: Verso.

Brennan, Claire. 2020. "Coronavirus: London Renting 'Feels Different' after Lockdown." *BBC News*. August 22, 2020. https://www.bbc.com/news/av/uk-england-london-53861413.

Butler, Judith. 2016. *Quadros de guerra: quando a vida é passível de luto*. 2nd ed. Translated by Sérgio Lamarão and Arnaldo Marques da Cunha. Rio de Janeiro: Civilização Brasileira.

Cabral, Diogo de Carvalho. 2014. *Na Presença da Floresta: Mata Atlântica e História Colonial*. Rio de Janeiro: Garamond/FAPERJ.

Carey, Mark. 2009. "Latin American Environmental History: Current Trends, Interdisciplinary Insights, and Future Directions." *Environmental History* 14, no. 2 (April): 221–52.

Conrad, Sebastian. 2016. *What is Global History?* Princeton: Princeton University Press.

Corbin, Alain. 1988. *Território do vazio: a praia e o imaginário Ocidental*. São Paulo: Companhia das Letras.

"Corona Paradise." 2021. *Corona Paradise*. 2021. https://www.coronaparadise.com.br/.

"Corona Paradise." 2023. *The Summer Hunter: We Follow the Sun*. 2023. https://thesummerhunter.com/brand/corona-paradise/.

Cronon, William. 1996. "The Trouble with Wilderness: Or, Getting Back to the Wrong Nature." *Environmental History* 1, no. 1: 7–28. https://doi.org/10.2307/3985059.

De Andrade, Oswaldo. 2009. *Pau Brasil*. Translated by Andrés Sánchez Robayna. Madrid: Fundación Juan March.

De Llano, Pablo. 2021. "La utopía urgente de volver al campo." *El País*. January 24, 2021. https://elpais.com/elpais/2021/01/20/eps/1611145093_375643.htm l.

Fairbairn, Madeleine, Jonathan Fox, S. R. Isakson, Michael Levien, Nancy Peluso, Shahra Razavi, Ian Scoones, and K. Sivaramakrishnan. 2014. "Introduction: New Directions in Agrarian Political Economy." *The Journal of Peasant Studies* 41, no. 5: 653–66. https://doi.org/10.1080/03066150.2014.953490.

"Fazenda da Grama." n.d. *Fazenda Da Grama*. Last accessed February 21, 2023. https://fazendadagrama.com.br/.

Fonseca, Caue. 2020. "Veranistas engrossam população do Litoral Norte durante a pandemia e cogitam mudanças em definitive." *GZH*. June 26, 2020. https://gauchazh.clicrbs.com.br/comportamento/noticia/2020/06/ veranistas-engrossam-populacao-do-litoral-norte-durante-a-pandemia-e-cogitam-mudancas-em-definitivo-ckbwmxpi30ohc0162ryoicjv6.html.

Freitag, Ulrike, and Achim von Oppen. 2010. "'Translocality': An Approach to Connection and Transfer in Area Studies." In *Translocality: The Study of Globalising Processes from a Southern Perspective*, edited by Ulrike Freitag and Achim von Oppen, 1–24. Leiden: Brill.

Freyre, Gilberto. (1933) 2011. *Casa-grande & senzala: Formação da família brasileira sobre o regime da economia patriarcal. Introdução à história da sociedade patriarcal no Brasil: Vol. 1*. 51. ed. São Paulo: Global Editora.

Graham, Stephen. 2016. *Cidades sitiadas. o novo urbanismo Militar*. São Paulo: Boitempo.

Howlett, Michael, and Rebecca Raglon. 1992. "Constructing the Environmental Spectacle: Green Advertisements and the Greening of the Corporate Image, 1910–1990." *Environmental History Review* 16, no. 4 (Winter): 53–68. http s://doi.org/10.2307/3984949.

Jauernig, Henning. 2021. "Wo das Haus im Grünen jetzt teurer wird." *Der Spiegel*. March 23, 2021. https://www.spiegel.de/wirtschaft/soziales/imm obilien-wo-das-haus-im-gruenen-jetzt-teurer-wird-a-9bbb96d6-11e4-41 67-a43d-b7fddc1b223f?sara_ecid=soci_upd_wbMbjhOSvViISjc8RPU89Nc CvtlFcJ.

Kaenzig, Raoul, and Etienne Piguet. 2011. "Migração e Mudança Climática na América Latina." *Revista Interdisciplinar da Mobilidade Humana* 19, no. 36: 49–74. https://www.redalyc.org/articulo.oa?id=407042013003.

Kaltmeier, Olaf. 2021. *National Parks from North to South: An Entangled History of Conservation and Colonization in Argentina*. New Orleans: University of New Orleans Press.

Lehmkuhl, Ursula, Hans-Jürgen Lüsebrink, and Laurence McFalls, eds. 2016. *Spaces of Difference: Conflicts and Cohabitation.* Münster: Waxmann.

Mbembe, Achille. 2016. "Necropolítica: biopoder, soberania, estado de exceção, política da morte." *Revista Arte e Ensaios 32* (December).

McNeill, J. R., and Erin Stewart Mauldin. 2012. "Global Environmental History: An Introduction." In *Wiley-Blackwell Companions to History: A Companion to Global Environmental History,* edited by J. R. McNeill and E. S. Mauldin, xvi–xxiv. New Jersey: Wiley-Blackwell.

Monzote, Reinaldo Funes. 2018. "The Greater Caribbean and the Transformation of Tropicality." In *A Living Past: Environmental Histories of Modern Latin America,* edited by John Soluri, Claudia Lael, and José Augusto Pádua, 46–66. New York: Berghahn.

Murari, Luciana. 2009. *Natureza e cultura no Brasil (1870–1922).* São Paulo: Alameda.

Nicolelis, Miguel A. L., Rafael L. G. Raimundo, Pedro S. Peixoto, and Cecilia S. Andreazzi. 2021. "The Impact of Super-Spreader Cities, Highways, and Intensive Care Availability in the Early Stages of the COVID-19 Epidemic in Brazil." *Scientific Reports* 11: 13001. https://doi.org/10.1038/1038/s41598-0 21-92263-3.

Noor, Farish A. 2020. "Crisis and Future: On the Demise of Dreams of Connectivity and Mobility." *TRAFO* (blog). November 6, 2020. https://trafo.hypoth eses.org/25434.

Pio, Juliana. 2020. "Neorrurais trocam cidade pelo campo em busca de novo estilo de vida." *Estadão.* September 20, 2020. https://www.estadao.com.b r/sustentabilidade/neorrurais-trocam-cidade-pelo-campo-em-busca-de-novo-estilo-de-vida/.

Ritter, Vivian Fetzner. 2014. "O espaço e a biopolítica." *Polietica* 2, no. 1: 112–37.

Ross, Corey. 2017. *Ecology and Power in the Age of Empire: Europe and the Transformation of the Tropical World.* Oxford: Oxford University Press.

Schossler, Joana Carolina. 2021. "Utopia balneária no Rio Grande do Sul: o mar como refúgio na Modernidade." *Percursos: Florianópolis* 22, no. 48: 430–55. h ttps://doi.org/10.5965/1984724622482021430.

Varnhagen, Francisco Adolfo de. 1870. *História geral do Brazil antes de sua separação e independência de Portugal.* 2nd ed. Rio de Janeiro: Laemmert.

Vieira, Patricia. 2018. *States of Grace: Utopia in Brazilian Culture.* New York: State University of New York Press.

Zweig, Stefan. (1941) 2013. *Brasilien—Ein Land der Zukunft.* Frankfurt am Main: Insel Verlag.

## Interviews

Caio Portugal. 2021. Brazilian Association of Subdivision and Urban Development Companies (Aelo). Interview by Danielle Heberle Viegas. October 8, 2021. Video. Transcription: Adriana Mastrangelo Ebecken.

Marcos Kathalian. Brain Institute: Strategic Intelligence. Interviewed by Danielle Heberle Viegas. October 6, 2021. Video. Transcription: Adriana Mastrangelo Ebecken.

Marina Figueiredo Braztoa. 2021. Brazilian Association of Tour Operators. Interviewed by Danielle Heberle Viegas. October 18, 2021. Video. Transcription: Adriana Mastrangelo Ebecken.

Pedro da Cunha e Menezes. 2021. Brazilian Trails Network. Interview by Danielle Heberle Viegas. October 5, 2021. Video. Transcription: Adriana Mastrangelo Ebecken.

Vinícius Viegas. 2021. Brazilian Ecotourism and Adventure Tourism Trade Association (ABETA). Interview by Danielle Heberle Viegas. October 21, 2021. Video. Transcription: Adriana Mastrangelo Ebecken.

# 8. Pandemic Play? Digital Sports Gaming, Fatness, and Contemporary Pandemic Imaginaries

*Martin Lüthe*

In an article published in the journal *Obesity Medicine* in September 2020, Moien AB Khan and Jane Elizabeth Moverley Smith identify a "new pandemic" as a result of the "behavioral, psychosocial, and environmental changes" brought about by the so-called lockdowns in response to the spread of COVID-19; they called this new pandemic "covibesity" (Khan and Smith 2020).[1] Khan and Smith and other researchers in medicine thus make use of the global spread of COVID-19 to shed light on another pandemic and the ways that the two kinds of pandemics seemed to be mutually reinforcing each other, namely COVID-19 and obesity. According to Khan, Smith and their peers, the research seems to suggest that COVID-19 cases might be more severe for patients who are also diagnosed as "obese," while the aforementioned lockdowns in response to COVID-19 increase the number of "obese" people in the world (due to an alleged lack of physical exercise) at the same time.

In the context of the current COVID-19 pandemic, then, complex discourses of health and physical vulnerability continue to take center stage, especially—if not only—in the form of the discursive proliferation of medical preconditions, risk groups, and what one might call the 'COVID/obesity' nexus under the rubric of public health. Recently, Nina Mackert and Friedrich Schorb have convincingly demonstrated how "public health, healthism, and fatness" intersect vehemently and how concerns over public health contribute powerfully to fat phobia. Considering the unwillingness for large-scale health reform, in the United States especially, "public health is increasingly occupied with the prevention of behavior that is presumed to induce health risks and

---

1    For similar arguments and findings, see for example: Santosh, Kumar KY, Praveen Kumar R Bhat, and Chandrashekar J Sorake. 2021. "Double Trouble: A Pandemic of Obesity and COVID-19."

its perceived outcomes such as fatness." The concerns over "covibesity" or the pandemic beneath the pandemic very much serve as reminders of how public health discourses and fat discourses frequently and powerfully intersect and have done so in the past (2022, 2).

In this chapter I approach pandemic imaginaries from a cultural studies' perspective. I am less interested in the medico-scientific truth value of pandemic connections, but in the cultural work the discourses of pandemics perform in our imaginaries and how they have become entangled with pervasive cultural anxieties pertaining to the digital age and its supposed impact on physical exercise and so-called abled bodies. My approach is grounded in disability studies in general and fat studies, specifically. At the core, I am interested in two types of bodies and how these embody pandemic imaginaries: The on-screen bodies and the off-screen bodies of digital games and digital sports games. These bodies signify what Lauren Berlant refers to as the 'crisis ordinary' of our age. Berlant situates the new aesthetics and genres she reads as defined by the affective attachments of "cruel optimism" in the 1990s and in the context of "a shift in how the older state-liberal-capitalist fantasies shape adjustments to the structural pressures of crisis" (2011, 7ff). At the same time, these shifts were accompanied by the transition towards digital home entertainment and coemerged with the success of the video gaming consoles. The so-called obesity pandemic, especially in U.S. and German public discourse, has frequently been linked to digital gaming as interrelated crises, often via the well disseminated insight that digital media use allegedly instills physical passivity in young people. Within the longer trajectory of historical discourses of media change, cultural critics and journalists have frequently analyzed the alleged connections between media use and the mental and physical health of young audiences as potentially dangerous as crucial elements of so-called media panics and as part of a discursive history of youth in crisis.[2]

Following a brief introduction of the fields of disability and fat studies, respectively, the chapter zooms in on the intersection of two discourses: namely the discourse of health/fitness and discourses of media change. I will briefly

---

2    For a longer history of cultural debates pertaining to the effects of media change on (young) audiences, see: Jeffrey Sconce. 2000. *Haunted Media*; Katherines Stubbs. 2004. "Telegraphy's Corporeal Fictions"; John Springhall. 1998. *Youth, Popular Culture and Moral Panics*; for a study of discourses of a youth in crisis and delinquency, see: Nina Mackert. 2014. "Danger and Hope: White Middle-Class Juvenile Delinquency and Parental Anxiety in the Postwar U.S."

analyze this discursive intersection in online news outlets in the U.S. and Germany to show how imaginations of the fatness pandemic and on digital gaming as a pandemic inform one another. I thus set out to enhance our understanding of the recent history of anxieties regarding body shape and so-called physical fitness. Arguably, these anxieties have recently intensified in the context of COVID-19, as the very notion of 'covibesity' indicates.

In the main analytical section of this contribution, I turn my attention to a recent example of the confluence of the two types of cultural concerns, health and media change, in the memes of so-called fat gamers or fat gamer kids. Memes, which the *Oxford Learner's Dictionary* defines as "an image, a video, a piece of text, etc. that is passed very quickly from one internet user to another, often with slight changes that make it humorous," have the capacity to condense and distill the meaning of specific cultural concepts and/or ideas into a single image (with a brief caption) ("Meme" n.d.).[3] I read the memes and the discourse of 'fat gamers' against the striking visual attention granted to the digital on-screen bodies of contemporary digital games. I seek to demonstrate that in-game 'bodies' frequently emerge as a problematic, as vulnerable sites, and that they thereby enter a meaningful relationship with the imagined body of the gamers opposite the interface. Arguably, these supposedly lazy, fat, gaming bodies themselves came to epitomize the cultural concerns pertaining to bodies stuck at home during the ongoing COVID-19 pandemic, of bodies slouching on couches and in front of the TV (and other screens) in our current pandemic imaginary.

Even before the lockdowns, however, the gaming bodies in front of the digital interface have begun to foreshadow the complexities of recent developments in our cultures of work: the digitization of work (from home) and its more recent 'zoomification' of the office. These allegedly inactive, fat bodies began to haunt the pandemic imaginary and have added to the discursive anxiety pertaining to our collective loss of 'fitness'; they thus amplify processes of othering of the 'fat gamer body' and of the 'fat Other' in general in our age of digitality. While the 'fat gamer' in the meme is clearly intended as the butt of the jokes, the memes also reveal an underlying anxiety regarding media change as such and media change as emblematic of changes in capitalist production

---

3    For an introduction to memes and a discussion of memes' capacity to encapsulate and communicate larger ideas, see: Eline Zenner and Dirk Geeraerts. 2018. "One Does Not Simply Process Memes: Image Macros as Multimodal Constructions."

thanks to digitization more generally. I utilize an intersectional lens to approach the memes and the tropes, because they clearly summon race, gender, age, and sexuality and thus might enable us to start comprehending the intersectional biopolitics of pandemic imaginaries, even as we seem to have—in June of 2022—collectively decided that the COVID-19 pandemic must be relegated to an imagined past.

## Disability Studies and Fat Bodies

In what follows I built on work at the nexus of critical feminist, queer and fat studies; as Marilyn Wann phrased it:

> In fat studies, there is respect for the political project of reclaiming the word *fat*, both as the preferred neutral adjective (i.e., short/tall, young/old, fat/thin) and also as preferred term of political identity. There is nothing negative or rude in the word fat unless someone makes the effort to put it there; using the word *fat* as a descriptor (not a discriminator) can help dispel prejudice. (2009, xii; emphasis in original)

Wann here outlines one of the crucial tenets of fat studies: Much like the projects of disability studies and queer studies, fat studies as a field sets out to make visible a pervasive cultural bias against marginalized groups and fat folks, specifically. In this sense, fat studies and disability studies enter a close conversation, because the anti-fat-bias circulating freely within and across the public and the medical discourses of our day (re)produces the ableist core principle of a healthy, functioning, (straight) human body as the central norm. As Rosemarie Garland-Thomson established in her programmatic text on "feminist disability studies":

> Feminist disability studies [similarly] questions our assumptions that disability is a flaw, lack, or excess. To do so, it defines disability broadly from a social rather than a medical perspective. Disability, it argues, is a cultural interpretation of human variation rather than an inherent inferiority, a pathology to cure, or an undesirable trait to eliminate. In other words, it finds disability's significance in interactions between bodies and their social and material environments. (2005, 1557)

Fatness as a category embodies all three of the assumptions listed by Garland-Thomson: a flaw, most notably in the way fat bodies are relegated to the side-lines and are largely made either invisible or become (freakishly) spectacular-ized in contemporary popular cultures in the Global North, in fashion, sports, and entertainment at large; the pseudo- and pop-medical discourses on fat-ness are frequently premised on the supposed lack of exercise and alleged lazi-ness of fat bodies, a process that has been further amplified by the abundance of health apps on our digital communication devices to monitor our activities, diets, and sleep; the excess of our current imaginaries of fat bodies center stage eating as practice, sweating, and, of course, the (fatness of the) flesh itself.[4] Additionally, however, fatness as a category is a spectrum; what that means is that there are different degrees to which people are read as, shamed as, or self-identify as "fat" (2005, 1557). Fatness is also intersectional, so every/body's experience varies according to the ways in which fatness intersects with other markers of social identity. It is thus not surprising that fatness is critically gen-dered and depictions of fat masculinities differ from how fatness intersects with femininities. As Daniel Farr writes in his introduction to a special issue of *Men and Masculinities*, "the being of any man, be he fat or thin, is influenced by the cultural politics of embodiment and weight; as there is no singular form of masculinity, there is no single form of fat masculinity" (2013, 384). Arguably, then, one of the pervasive forms of fat masculinity in our time intersects with the stereotype of the computer geek and/or the gamer addict. Cultural arti-facts and opinion pieces abound that express concern (or make fun of) lonely men in their 'man caves' who refuse to grow up, who are socially unreliable, who get addicted to the games they play and pose a problem in their relation-ships by withdrawing from life in 'the real world' altogether. These depictions of fat, lonely men evoke the pervasive media cultural practice of marking non-hegemonic masculinities as deviant and undesirable. Fatness here, along with media addiction, serve as signifiers of a deviant, non-hegemonic, less virile version of masculinity.[5]

---

4    For a discussion of the relationship between fat studies and disability studies, see: Rosemarie Garland-Thomson. 2005. "Feminist Disability Studies"; Anna Mollow. 2017. "Disability Studies Gets Fat."

5    As an example of the male gaming addict as journalistic trope, see: Tanya J. Peterson. 2021. "My Husband Is Addicted to Gaming: You're Not Alone." For more on hegemonic and non-hegemonic masculinities, see: R.W. Connell. 1983. *Which Way Is Up? Essays on Sex and Culture*; R.W. Connell & James W. Messerschmidt. 2005. "Hegemonic Masculin-ity: Rethinking the Concept."

Even those articles that approach the topic of gaming addiction with the help of experts and a seemingly open catalogue of questions, frequently utilize menacing visuals to prime their readers regarding the inherent dangers of gaming and the potentially debilitating effects of gaming on young men's mental and physical health. Ferris Jabr's article, "Can You Really Be Addicted to Video Games?", published in *New York Times Magazine* on October 22, 2019, features a prominent visual on top, which only displays a PS4 Dual Sense controller positioned in the middle of a bright yellow surface. The isolated device, the controller, is plastered with warning stickers (e.g.: "Use With Caution") and thus communicates a sense of isolation, loneliness, and imminent danger. The question posed as the title to the piece, "Can You Really Be Addicted to Video Games?", seems to be prematurely answered by the image selected to introduce the article. The image of the sole controller is powerful in that it makes us as readers imagine who the intended audience is for such warnings. Now picture that person: he is male, he is young-ish, you probably picture him as white, and in your mind he is probably fat. Even if the journalistic images of gamers do not exclusively depict men who are fat, many articles and outlets contextualize stock images of gamers and gaming with explicit or implicit references to the disabling fatness of some of the gamers.

The German news outlet *Spiegel Online*, for example, similarly deployed a head visual of the 'lonely controller' in an article warning about the video gaming/fatness nexus in 2017. Additionally, however, the article used the visual framing of the single controller only to deliver a stunning first paragraph on the potentially detrimental effects of digital gaming on young boys: "Maurice war ein normaler Schüler, als er mit sieben seine erste Playstation bekam. Der Junge spielte gern damit, aber noch ging die Schule vor. In der sechsten Klasse fing er an, auch mal krankzumachen. Er hockte daheim vorm Bildschirm, aß Kartoffelchips, trank Cola und wurde dick." (Maurice was a normal student, when he got his first Playstation at age 7. The boy enjoyed playing with it, but school still came first. In the 6th grade he started playing hooky [pretending to be sick]. He sat at home eating potato chips, drinking coke, and got fat) ("Was übertriebener Medienkonsum" 2017; my translation).[6] While I find it hard to contest the article's general call to raise awareness regarding media use and media literacy, describing the seeming unraveling of a boy's life in four short sentences at the beginning of an article undoubtedly runs the risk

---

6    For a similar example in a different outlet in Germany, see Thomas Lindemann. 2008. "Videospiele machen schlau—und fett."

of dramatically simplifying the complex processes at work in any person's life. Also, of course, the article makes use of the triad of 'eating potato chips, drinking coke' and 'getting fat' to describe a process at the end of which the boy serves only as a warning for an alarmed (assumed) readership.

Arguably, then, these and similar examples, published in news outlets and across the web, set the stage for some of our current anxieties regarding the spread of 'Covibesity.' What is more, however, these news reports on gaming circulate through media environments that add to and amplify the alleged scandalous 'fat gamers' that video gaming produces. The fat gamer memes, after all, condense this anxious discourse regarding off-screen fatness captured in the opening sentences to the *Spiegel Online* piece, as this stereotype—deployed frequently in reporting on gaming in mainstream outlets—finds its viral expression on the web in the form of a meme, simply called the fat gamer meme.

## The On-Screen-Fitness/Off-Screen Fatness Binary and 'Two Pandemics'

The standard foil for the fat gamer meme features the face of a fat white teenager with an unkempt (half-shaven) beard, a pimpled face, glasses, and a ponytail in front of a multicolored background. Above his face we find, in white printed letters, the set-up to joke and below the face its punchline. These are premised on the unattractiveness and/or the unworldliness of the depicted gamer. "'Outside' ... Never Heard of That Server" or "Got back together with my ex ... xbox360" serve as typical examples of the meme and of how it operates. The images selected here show the template of the meme, the color scheme, and the arrangement of the joke (fig. 4 and fig. 5):

*Figure 4:* Fat Gamer Meme *taken from quickmeme.com.*

*Figure 5:* Fat Gamer Meme *taken from Imgflip.com.*

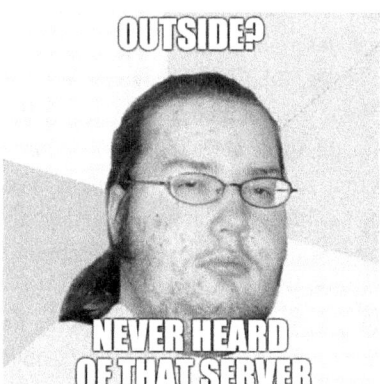
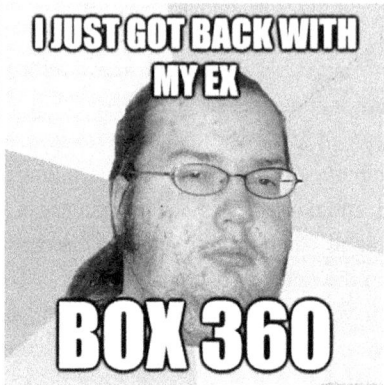

The meme template consists of a square broken up into six brightly colored tiles, a neon green one, two more or less neon red ones, and three variations of orange. At the heart of these tiles we find a close-up of a pimpled, bespectacled, fat face of a young man, who has his greasy hair pulled back in a pony-tail. The top of the meme features the set-up of the joke in big white capital letters and below the image of the 'fat gamer' the meme displays the punch-line in the same, simple style.

The variations of the meme are obviously premised on a cliched notion of video game cultures and individuals playing games. Crucially, these images and the jokes establish a close connection between 'fatness' and gaming, between an unhealthy diet and a lack of physical activity engrained into gaming culture and a withdrawal from life beyond the digital interfaces. Additionally, the visuals and the jokes taken together establish a white, male, youngish, fat gaming Other and the memes frequently poke fun at the fat gamer's alleged ignorance of anything outside of the practices and lore of gaming culture. Arguably, the memes distill an entire discourse about digital cultures and the bodies (and minds) of young (white) men into images and punchlines and thereby underscore the importance and the truth claims of the journalistic discourse exemplified above. Frequently, the memes' jokes also underscore the heteronormativity of the discourses of health they are a part of, as they center-stage the fat gamer's sexual inexperience and his lack of interest in (hetero)sexual intercourse or romantic relationships. This sheds light on two crucial ways in which the memes mark their tragic protagonist as deviant: Firstly, the memes double-down on the assumed unattractiveness of the image of the fat gamer by additionally branding him as essentially asexual; secondly, by establishing the absence of the fat gamer's heteronormative desire to have sex (or to bond romantically) the memes naturalize the alleged interconnection between heterosexual reproductivity and physical and mental health that has historically served as a cornerstone of social and cultural constructions of hegemonic masculinities. As a consequence, fatness and gaming co-emerge as the undesirable Other of these constructions of hegemonic masculinities. Additionally, the trope of the unattractive and asexual gamer marks him as explicitly undesirable and without desires of himself (beyond gaming) and thus further alludes to common discourses of the effects of addiction at large. Also, the heteronormative framework and the absent vectors of desire contribute to dis-easing the fat gamer and to other him as decisively—physically and mentally—unhealthy. It is in these processes of the naturalization of the fat gamer as unhealthy and effeminate Other that the memes foreshadowed the discursive and biopolitical investment in the health of the body politic in the context of the COVID-19 pandemic.

This investment in the imagined off-screen bodies of fat gamers finds its mirror image in the in-game representation of physically fit and excelling bodies, especially but not only in contemporary digital sports games, such as the FIFA, Madden, NBA 2K, or PES franchises (now called efootball). As Ella Brians reminds us: "Historically, cyber discourses have been characterized by a desire to transcend the perceived limits of materiality, which inevitably means transcending the body" and that "while versions of cyber discourse that argue for taking embodiment seriously have emerged, the fantasy of escaping the flesh persists" (2011, 118). At the same time, however, digital sports games deal with bodily complexities in a different manner, as they redirect our attention to the in-game bodies as crucial sites which are intended to embody the 'realistic' potentials and limits of the bodies of professional athletes. The bodies' movements on the virtual playing field, the impact of physical contact and interaction between players, and the range of creating soccer and American football players' bodies in the edit modes of both games have been improved from year to year. Not surprisingly then, both franchises have frequently marketed recent releases by also explicitly advocating the improved production of the physical body of the players in the game. As a consequence, these games frequently reproduce specific kinds of racialized fantasies pertaining to the professional athletes' male bodies as part of their editing and gaming modes (see also Leonard 2005).

Whereas the reproduction of ideologies of gender and race intersect in the games' deployment of physicality, it is the production of the body in the game's core element of gameplay that is most complex. Evidently, sports are dependent on a specific utilization of physical expertise and while the significance of the mind in soccer, for example for the realm of tactics and analyzing an opponent, can and have been simulated with an astonishing degree of realism, certain physical aspects of the game seem still harder to simulate. For digital sports games this arguably provides the most problematic part regarding an actual simulation of real-world sports; as Andrew Baerg argues, both optimistic and pessimistic discourses regarding the (ir)relevancy of the physical body for digital sports gaming are of importance for the cultural study of digital gaming, and "these kinds of discourses become important to consider in thinking about the material nature of bodies in real-world sport as they become translated into new media and how this translation shapes the experience of sport" (2007, 329).

Accordingly, it is the in-between and the process of translating real-life and digital gaming experiences of physicality—back and forth—that provide the most critical potential for fruitful analyses of corporeality and/in digital gaming. The on-screen, on-field bodies emerge as vulnerable sites, however, particularly at those moments, when the games aspire to simulate injuries in-game. For much of film history, maimed male bodies provided Hollywood movies with their quintessential visual language to invoke an alleged crisis of masculinity, idealized as able-bodied, as athletic, as virile. As, for example, Susan Jeffords has argued, the long history of the depiction of wounded male bodies, for example in Hollywood war movies, has provided U.S. culture with a register to metonymically depict a perceived crisis of masculinity on the silver screen that the hypermasculine title—giving 1980s—"hard bodies" of her study provided a filmic response to (cf. 1994, 11ff.).[7]

Similarly, digital sports games have represented injuries and pain with a continuously increasing attention to detail, often by simulating the broadcasting strategy of instant replays and/or through filmic intermissions in so-called cut scenes. Instant replays in sports gaming as well as in televised sports narratively structure the event at hand. Arguably, the broadcasting director's decisions of which scene demands or deserves instant replays could be regarded as his or her central concern and his/her most powerful tool to impact how the

---

7    For a discussion of the relationship between the games and gamers, see also: Nate Garrelts, "Introduction: Negotiating the Digital Game/Gamer Intersection."

television audience perceives a televised sports event; accordingly, the same holds true for the programmers and producers of digital sports games, for example of EA's FIFA series or Konami's Pro Evolution Soccer franchise (which has recently been revamped as eFootball in 2022). The filmic sequences of an in-game player writhing that digital soccer games deploy simulates the real-life sports practice of players performing pain in order to increase the likeability for referees to implement draconian measures against the offender on the one hand; on the other hand, the sequences of players in pain keep the gamer in suspense as to whether or not the player can continue playing or needs to be substituted as a result of an injury. If the on-screen player was mildly injured, he can continue to play, even though his physical abilities are noticeably impeded and the sequence of a subsequent substitution of the player will show him limp of the field, his face contorted with pain.[8]

There are at least two ways to conceive of the connection between the visual attention granted to injured players on screen and the off-screen bodies of the (fat) gamer: Firstly and superficially, these cut-scenes serve the purpose to create and recreate the appearance and appeal of the live sports broadcast audiences are familiar with. Secondly, however, something else appears to be at stake, when we move those bodies swiftly across the pitch and then they get stopped rigorously and painfully by opposing defenders; namely the very vulnerability of bodies as such and of virile, male bodies specifically. Here, the conventionalized split between the body before and the body on the interface makes itself felt and emerges as a problematic of our digital age. We find that split between the athletic, hegemonic male body of the digital sport game and the presumably slouching, passive body of the gamer hardly anywhere more pronounced than in digital sports gaming. As I have delineated, the tropes of the deviant, fat, gaming body of the digital age have recently begun to inform discourses about youths (and the generation of digital natives) in the United States and Western Europe, especially in the context of an alleged decline in real-life athletic abilities. Thus, the trope of the male injured body in digital

8    For a discussion of physicality and the representation of bodies in digital sports games, see: Andrew Baerg. "Fight Night Round 2: Mediating the Body and Digital Boxing"; see also Lüthe, Martin. "2013. "(Re-)producing the Body: Motion Capture and the Meaning of Physicality in Digital Soccer Games"; for a general history of digital sports games, see: Andrew Baerg. "It's in the Game: The History of Sports Video Games"; for a general history of digital games, see: Lucien King. *Game On: The History and Culture of Video Games*; also: Carroll Pursell. *From Playgrounds to Playstation: The Interaction of Technology and Play.*

sports games—along with the fat gamer memes—contribute to a current discourse over the 'gaming body' of our times. In an almost paradoxical manner,
these young, athletic, male bodies on the screen make our current anxieties
vis-à-vis a generation of supposedly fat bodies off-screen visible; partly via the
imagined juxtaposition and partly at moments of game-flow disruption: at the
very moments on-screen bodies become injured in the digital sports simula-
tions and thus make tangible the very fragility of those male, athletic bodies we
deem hegemonically masculine on and off the screen.

## (In lieu of a) Conclusion

At its core, the fat gamer memes expose an inherent tension in our neoliberal
late-capitalist and media-capitalist fantasies regarding economic productivity
and the bodies that perform them with the help of machines and algorithms:
on the one hand, capitalism cherishes the inventors, programmers, and experts of the digital now, on the other hand we demonize the imagined bodies of
fat gaming nerds as deviant and unhealthy. The memes only manage to thinly
veil the angst they capture regarding the future of the labor force of digital capitalism as an expression of anxieties regarding the future of capitalist productivity as such; and like earlier discourses on a younger generation in/as crisis
in historic moments of pervasive media change, the memes connect the health
and well-being of a younger generation on the level of the individual young
gamer, as a pandemic of individual weakness, not, for example, as an outcome
of the privatization of public goods, such as health insurance and health services in general. And because it concerns the kids, like Maurice, it is always
already about the future.

I do not intend to deny the challenge of media education for our generation
and those to come, but the fervor and anxiety with which the discourse works
to establish a 'fat gaming Other' evokes a long history of articulations of cultural anxieties regarding those of us who have been deemed 'unproductive': the
lazy, the drunk, the addicted, the young delinquents, the drifters of our capitalist imaginaries. It is in this sense that the meme provides a discursive ac-
complice to the trope of the pained male on-screen body with its long tradition
in our cultural imaginaries. Put differently: the fat gamer continues the ways
in which media have represented the dis/abled binary and their ableist agenda
by connecting it to socio-economic (and erotic) 'productivity.' The fat gamer
meme—as a mirror image to the injured male body of the Hollywood film of

earlier—continues a tradition of representation for our digital and pandemic now, as it also unmasks our overall anxiety regarding digital culture(s) and the potential experts of our new age (i.e. an age of digital work, zoomification, and big data). Sadly, as we collectively have wished COVID away in 2022 and early 2023, the cultural anxiety pertaining to fatness and the 'pandemic beneath the pandemic' of course are here to stay, as our health app keep us conscious of our weight and exercise (or lack thereof) and if we were to collectively or individually ignore them, the memes will do their work to keep us alert about the inherent dangers of 'letting ourselves go' in front of the abundant screens of our lives.

## Works Cited

Baerg, Andrew. 2007. "Fight Night Round 2: Mediating the Body and Digital Boxing." *Sociology of Sport Journal* 24, no. 3 (September): 325–45.

———. 2013. "It's in the Game: The History of Sports Video Games." In vol. 2 of *American History through American Sports: From Colonial Lacrosse to Extreme Sports*, edited by Danielle Sarver Coombs and Bob Batchelor, 75–90. Westport: Praeger.

Berlant, Lauren. 2011. *Cruel Optimism*. Durham: Duke University Press.

Brians, Ella. 2011. "The 'Virtual' Body and the Strange Persistence of the Flesh: Deleuze, Cyberspace and the Posthuman." In *Deleuze and the Body*, edited by Laura Guillaume and Joe Hughes, 117–43. Edinburgh: Edinburgh University Press.

Connell, R. W. 1983. *Which Way Is Up? Essays on Sex and Culture*. Sydney: Allen and Unwin.

Connell, R. W., and James W. Messerschmidt. 2005. "Hegemonic Masculinity: Rethinking the Concept." *Gender and Society* 19, no. 6: 829–59.

Farr, Daniel. 2013. "Introduction to the Special Issue: Fat Masculinities." *Men and Masculinities* 16, no. 4 (October): 383–6.

"Fat Gamer Meme: I'm Going to See my Ex Xbox." n.d. *Imgflip*. Last Accessed March 2, 2023. https://imgflip.com/meme/16500471/fat-gamer.

"Fat Gamer Meme: Outside? Never Heard of That Server." n.d. *Quick Meme*. Last Accessed March 2, 2023. http://www.quickmeme.com/meme/30pfjv.

"Fat Gamer Meme Template." n.d. *Imgflip*. Last Accessed March 2, 2023. https://imgflip.com/memetemplate/16500471/fat-gamer.

Garland-Thomson, Rosemarie. 2005. "Feminist Disability Studies." *Signs: Journal of Women in Culture and Society* 30, no. 2 (Winter): 1557–87.

Garrelts, Nate. 2005. "Introduction: Negotiating the Digital Game/Gamer Intersection." In *Digital Gameplay: Essays on the Nexus of Game and Gamer*, edited by Nate Garrelts, 1–19. Jefferson: McFarland.

Jabr, Ferris. 2019. "Can You Really Be Addicted to Video Games?" *New York Times Magazine*. October 22, 2019. https://www.nytimes.com/2019/10/22/magazine/can-you-really-be-addicted-to-video-games.html.

Jeffords, Susan. 1994. *Hard Bodies: Hollywood Masculinity in the Reagan Era*. New Brunswick: Rutgers University Press.

Khan, Moien A.B., and Elizabeth Moverley Smith. 2020. "'Covibesity,' a New Pandemic." *Obesity Medicine* 19, (September). https://doi.org/10.1016/j.obmed.2020.100282.

King, Lucien. 2008. *Game On: The History and Culture of Video Games*. London: Laurence King.

Leonard, David J. 2005. "To the White Extreme: Conquering Athletic Space, White Manhood, and Racing Virtual Reality." In *Digital Gameplay: Essays on the Nexus of Game and Gamer*, edited by Nate Garrelts, 110–28. Jefferson: McFarland.

Lindemann, Thomas. 2008. "Videospiele machen schlau—und Fett." *Die Welt*. August 20, 2008. https://www.welt.de/wirtschaft/webwelt/article2325745/Videospiele-machen-schlau-und-fett.html.

Lüthe, Martin. 2013. "(Re-)producing the Body: Motion Capture and the Meaning of Physicality in Digital Soccer Games." In *Build 'em Up—Shoot 'em Down: Körperlichkeit in Digitalen Spielen*, edited by Peter Just and Rudolf Inderst, 25–41. Glückstadt: Werner Hülsbusch.

Mackert, Nina. 2014. "Danger and Hope: White Middle-Class Juvenile Delinquency and Parental Anxiety in the Postwar U.S." In *Juvenile Delinquency and Western Modernity, 1800–2000*, edited by Heather Ellis, 199–224. New York: Palgrave Macmillan.

Mackert, Nina, and Friedrich Schorb. 2022. "Introduction to the Special Issue: Public Health, Healthism, and Fatness." *Fat Studies* 11, no. 1 (January): 1–7. https://doi.org/10.1080/21604851.2021.1911486.

"Meme." n.d. *Oxford Learner's Dictionary*. Last Accessed June 21, 2022. https://www.oxfordlearnersdictionaries.com/definition/english/meme.

Mollow, Anna. 2015. "Disability Studies Gets Fat." *Hypatia* 30, no. 1: 199–216.

Peterson, Tanya J. 2021. "My Husband Is Addicted to Gaming: You're Not Alone." *Healthy Place*. December 15, 2021. https://www.healthyplace.co

m/addictions/gaming-disorder/my-husband-is-addicted-to-gaming-you
re-not-alone.

Pursell, Carroll. 2015. *From Playgrounds to Playstation: The Interaction of Technology and Play*. Baltimore: Johns Hopkins University Press.

Santosh, Kumar KY, Praveen Kumar R. Bhat, and Chandrashekar J. Sorake. 2021. "Double Trouble: A Pandemic of Obesity and COVID-19." *The Lancet: Gastroenterology & Hepatology* 6, no. 8 (August). https://doi.org/10.1016/S246 8-1253(21)00190-4.

Sconce, Jeffrey. 2000. *Haunted Media: Electronic Presence from Telegraphy to Television*. Durham: Duke University Press.

Springhall, John. 1998. *Youth, Popular Culture and Moral Panics: Penny Gaffs to Gangsta-Rap, 1830–1996*. London: Palgrave Macmillan.

Stubbs, Katherine. 2004. "Telegraphy's Corporeal Fictions." In *New Media, 1740–1915*, edited by Lisa Gitelman and Geoffrey B. Pingree, 91–112. Cambridge: MIT Press.

Wann, Marilyn. 2009. "Foreword: Fat Studies; An Invitation to Revolution." In *The Fat Studies Reader*, edited by Esther Rothblum and Sondra Soloway, ix–xxv. New York: New York University Press.

"Was übertriebener Medienkonsum bei Ihrem Kind anrichten kann." 2017. *Spiegel Wissenschaft*. November 12, 2017. https://www.spiegel.de/spiegel/i nternetsucht-und-fettleibigkeit-was-kinder-ins-unglueck-treibt-a-11774 64.html.

Zenner, Eline, and Dirk Geeraerts. 2018. "One Does Not Simply Process Memes: Image Macros as Multimodal Constructions." In *Cultures and Traditions of Wordplay and Wordplay Research*, edited by Esme Winter-Froemel and Verena Thaler, 167–93. Berlin: De Gruyter.

# 9. The Virus Is Present, Presence Is Virulent: Being Co(m)present with Others in Times of the COVID-19 Pandemic

*Julia Eckel and Elisa Linseisen*

This contribution starts from the observation that the main challenge of a pandemic situation is the problem of presence[1] which, simultaneously, is a central problem of media(lity) (Keidl et al. 2020). Presence—basically understood as the idea of a spatial and temporal concurrent state of being—has become one of the most important issues under 'pandemic conditions' because it reveals itself as the central problem and at the same time as a necessity which is sought to be achieved and ensured through the use of media. As Helen Parish (2020) states, a pandemic condition is characterized by "the absence of presence and the presence of absence," and therefore by a strong need to (re)define what presence means and what it means to be present. In short: When a virus is present, presence becomes virulent.

In a pandemic, being physically (co-)present with someone else entails the danger of contagion. It thus requires forms of 'social distancing' which lead to an increase in media usage as a (para)social substitute (telephones, video conferences, voice mails, etc.). At the same time, the invisibility of the virus itself necessitates that it is 'made present'—meaning: in a mediated form (through numbers, graphs, CGI, talking heads of politicians and experts, etc.). Therefore, it seems that the first strategy to prevent the virus from spreading is to fight its potential presence in human bodies by means of a presence of human bodies in media. As physical *copresence* vanishes, alternative, inevitably mediated types, of presence come into focus, which we want to explore with the help of the complementary term *compresence*.

---

1   We want to thank Leonie Zilch for many fruitful discussions we had on the topic of (mediated) presence and for all her thoughts and ideas that she shared with us and that found their way into this paper.

Building on these ideas, a pandemic condition could be conceived as a framework in which presence as a concept and phenomenon needs to be problematized and where it (re-)constitutes itself in relation to media. What presence means under these circumstances can be assessed, firstly, in terms of its mediated spatio-temporality, which marks a kind of 'shift' from the idea of immediate (co-)presence to the complex relationship of distance and proximity linked to "mediated presence" (Spagnolli et al. 2009). And secondly, another level of reference is irritated by this shift, one that complements space and time. This is the differentiation of public and private, which correlates with the constitution of the self in difference to (an)other and which, as we will show, generates modes of othering. Our aim is to counter these structures of differentiation with the idea of compresence, a term that raises notions of togetherness and community and also allows to analyze the pandemic impact on a media theoretical understanding of presence.

Hence, the article explores two interrelated assumptions: 1) that the so-called 'corona crisis' is accompanied by a crisis of *copresence* that manifests itself mainly in forms of othering and 2) that this crisis is additionally strongly related to media which brings aspects of *compresence* to the fore. Our argument is that the differentiation of *copresence* and *compresence*, as two not binary but intertwined tendencies of presence, helps to identify precarious as well as productive intersections between media, knowledge, society, and the individual that become especially visible and virulent during pandemic times but apply to general societal structures as well. Although our findings focus primarily on the COVID-19 pandemic and are situated within European and North American contexts, some of the results might nevertheless be transferable to pandemics in general.

## (Mediated) Presence and Othering

Presence is one of the most central aspects of media as the question of mediality is centered around phenomena of (re)production and therefore the (re)*present*ation of things and events (Benjamin [1935] 2013; Derrida 2003; Gumbrecht 2003 and 2014; Kiening 2007; Spagnolli et al. 2009; Ernst and Paul 2013). Practices of mediation constitute, simulate, and negotiate presence. Hence, media studies draw on a large number of heterogeneous inter- and transdisciplinary theories about the impact of media(ted) presence on culture and society.

From a media historical perspective, for example, the current pandemic condition, its structure and mediality, can be better understood by comparing it to other turning points in the media theoretical concept of presence: Out of the multitude of examples from the history of media that have led to key questions of media theory, let us only briefly mention a few developments, e.g. the rise of *privacy* during the eighteenth century when Western cultures saw an increase of alphabetization and the growth of postal infrastructures, leading to literate substitutions of physical presence (love letters, diaries, etc.) and a new concept of intimacy (Siegert 1993).[2] This medial form of closeness in distance seemed to allow for a potentiation of presence. Another example is the emergence of *tele-communication* and *liveness*, which is strongly linked to the advent of technological mass media (radio, television, etc.) in the twentieth century (McLuhan 2001). These dimensions have been widely discussed in media theory, for example under the term "telepresence," first formally used by the AI-scientist Marvin Minsky (1980), describing the ability and benefits to remote-control things. Again, in these cases presence seems to develop new agencies and qualities through media, which in television studies are directly linked to the quality of the medial image itself (Bracken 2005) and lead to the exploration of new forms of embodiment as an opportunity for feminist, queer, and crip media theoretical approaches (Foster 1997; Haden 2015). But with digitalization on the horizon, forms of mediated presence at the end of the twentieth century are also perceived as a cause for criticism in postmodern theorizations, because presence is suspected of simulation and suspended by hyperrealism and virtual reality (Virilio 1991).

As prominent as the question of presence therefore is in media studies, it has not been related to pandemic situations in terms of media history and media theory so far. If the pandemic is the extreme case of a precarization of presence, the lack of media theoretical discussions of the term seems rather unusual. As we have experienced during the COVID-19 pandemic, when media practices (e.g. video conferences) undergo an increase in relevance compared to other communicative practices (e.g. information transfer through 'office grapevine'), this shift implies political dimensions which bring up broader questions of (re)presentation, such as: How do currently privileged media practices or representations manifest or subvert existing social and political

---

2    For a re-evaluation of the concept of intimacy in times of digital media see e.g. Cefai and Couldry 2019.

structures? How are issues of class, race, gender, (dis)ability, or age (re)pro-
duced through media practices? Who speaks, i.e. who gets 'screen time' and
is consequently present or not? Some of these issues—like the decrease of
submitted papers from female scientists due to (child)care duties (Bowyer et
al. 2021) but also the struggles of childfree women in academia (França 2022),
the presence of virologists as mostly male identified experts during the crisis,
or the presentation of female identified nurses and supermarket workers as
'systematically relevant' (Milan et al. 2021; Dudley 2022)—are already discussed and researched. Who or what is or can be (re)presented in the media
draws boundaries and thereby produces and distributes a present and an
absent, an (in)visible and an (in)audible, noise and information. With Jacques
Rancière (2004), we want to speak here of the division of the sensual as an
explicitly political concern. During the COVID-19 pandemic these social and
political boundaries and borders have become exponentially virulent and even
more complex because the difference between the individual and the social,
the body and the state collapses. As Paul Preciado (2020) resumes in his critical
essay "Learning from the Virus," which analyzes the nexus of community and
immunity in relation to the border politics of Europe and the USA:

> The body, your individual body, as a life space and as a network of power,
> as a center of production and of energy consumption, has become the new
> territory where the violent border politics that we have been designing and
> testing for years on 'others' are now expressed, now taking the form of con-
> tainment measures and of a war against the virus. The new necropolitical
> frontier has shifted from the coast of Greece toward the door of your home.
> Lesbos now starts at your doorstep. And the border is forever tightening
> around you, pushing you ever closer to your body. Calais blows up in your
> face. The new frontier is the mask. The air that you breathe has to be yours
> alone. The new frontier is your epidermis. The new Lampedusa is your skin.
> For years, we considered migrants and refugees infectious to the commu-
> nity and placed them in detention centers – political limbos where they re-
> mained without rights and without citizenship; perpetual waiting rooms.
> Now we are living in detention centers in our own homes.

Referring to COVID-19 as the "invisible other," as Annamaria Silvana de
Rosa and Terri Mannarini (2021) have done, and assuming that everyone is
potentially infected—the "invisible other" from whom one must distance
oneself—we pursue the question of how media presence produces forms of
othering in the context of the pandemic. 'Pandemic othering' refers not only

to the demarcation of boundaries between individuals and 'other' entities, but also shapes the (self-)perception of the individual. As Yvonne Zimmermann (2020) has argued in relation to phenomena of self-perception as self-othering in software like Zoom, "videoconferencing has brought about a new relationship of closeness and distance of self and/as other. It is an uncanny encounter, a self-reflection as imaged self/other that opens up to a specific mode of self-reflexivity: to self-monitoring 2.0" (Zimmermann 2022, 99). However, going beyond de Rosa and Mannarini's spatio-cultural analysis and Zimmermann's focus on 'the self' and 'the other' as a personal relation, we want to explicitly address the discriminatory and (post-)colonial moments of othering that occur in processes of distancing oneself through mediated presence. For example, Minsky's concept of telepresence rests on the idea of a simulation of proximity that promises the ability to handle and control objects from a distance. This means, in a literal sense, that telepresence is redeemed for Minsky by the robotic hand that brings distance within reach: "Using this instrument, you can 'work' in another room, in another city, in another country, or on another planet. Your remote presence possesses the strength of a giant or the delicacy of a surgeon. Heat or pain is translated into informative but tolerable sensation. Your dangerous job becomes safe and pleasant" (1980, 45). Even if the techno-utopia that Minsky sketches in 1980 does not address the military and imperial applications of remote control, this dimension of technology is certainly present in the idea of mediated presence through the control of the 'other' from the safety and comfort of the 'own.' Mediated presence in this sense seems to serve only to establish a sovereign subject that designates 'others' as such in order to constitute itself as an acting, operating sovereign. This, as Gayatri Chakravorty Spivak explains in detail, corresponds exactly to the European strategy of establishing and administering colonies by force (1985). The term 'othering' names various strategies by which colonial discourse produces its subjects, and postcolonial media theory shows that these strategies are medial, as they (audio)visually, iconographically, narratively and epistemologically produce and represent an imperial logic and 'truth' of the colonized world (Fernández 1999; Bergermann and Heidenreich 2015; Merten and Krämer 2016). As Spivak shows, othering is a dialectical process, mutually constituting the colonizing Other (with capital "O," the sovereign) and the colonized others.[3] This process of binary separation, which violently legit-

---

3    In many theories of (post-)colonialism, this differentiation by capitalization of the 'O' is used the other way around which means that the discriminated and marginalized

imizes the hegemony, 'virtue,' and 'naturalness' of the colonizing culture, can be directly linked to forms of mediated presence. During pandemic times and beyond, media(ted) presence not only (re)produces social/political processes of othering, but it does so as a process of aesthetic/technological othering, in the sense of Rancière's theory cited above. Cultural processes of othering are, in this sense, initiated by and inextricably linked to media presence.

It is precisely through the apparent paradox of a mediated presence that the relationship between self and Other becomes virulent in its complexity. The postcolonial theoretical concept of othering helps us to examine this complex relationship of mediated presence in terms of its power mechanisms. This is particularly relevant since new forms of vulnerability and also of violence emerge in digital space.[4] Hence, we offer the following preliminary conclusion: Media presence produces powerful moments of othering in the complex interweaving of near and far, own and Other. We now want to ask to what extent these discriminatory tendencies can be countered or to what extent there are possibilities for a media presence beyond this violent power structure. To this end, we propose the concept of compresence.

---

group is referred to by the term 'Other(s)' – in opposition to 'the self' or 'the own' that usually depicts a *white* (and most of the time male) Western colonizer. In both ways, the 'O' is used to mark the term as an instrument of power established by the colonizing force. Although we refer to Spivak's theory here, we will nevertheless follow the convention of this book to use the term 'Others' with capital O for the colonized (see the introduction by Heike Steinhoff, n6). When we use the term 'other' with lower-case O it shall mark contexts where we are not speaking about colonized or marginalized subjects but other self-defining relations. For further reading on the term of 'the Other' in postcolonial theory see also Ashcroft, Griffiths and Tiffin 2007, 154–6.

4    In the context of the *Forum Antirassismus Medienwissenschaft*, which was founded during the pandemic by media scholars from German-speaking countries across statuses and locations, a handout was created that draws attention to violent moments of othering, especially in digital settings such as Zoom rooms, e.g., in relation to visibilities. In addition to the undeniably sexist and racist attacks of so-called Zoom bombing, the simple question of who turns on the camera in a Zoom room and who does not, can lead to a colonization of the seemingly neutral digital space: "A concomitant phenomenon is that the new visibilities and openings of interaction spaces that accompany digitalization create new vulnerabilities that can be exploited by different actors with different motivations." (Eickelmann et al. 2021, 1; translated by Elisa Linseisen; see also Nunes and Ozog 2021).

## From Copresence to Compresence

Looking at the *Merriam Webster Dictionary* the difference between 'copresence' and 'compresence' lies in the quality of the type of presence. While "copresence" means the "occurrence of two or more things together in the same place and time" (n.d.) and thus focuses more on physical qualities in a spatio-temporal continuum, the word "compresence" is translated as "the quality or state of being present together" (n.d.)—which seems to focus more on an abstract form of 'togetherness.' We want to use this difference in meaning between copresence and compresence, and especially the emphasis on the shared, relational nature of compresence, productively to show the potentials of media presence during a pandemic. The idea is to complement and counteract otherness with togetherness. In this respect, we understand compresence as a way of describing new forms of medial commonality in times of precarious sociality. The pandemic represents an extreme situation in this respect, but it has only made pre- and post-pandemic social structures visible in an exaggerated way.

In this sense, the notion of compresence points to an alternative to the violent dimensions of othering that a media presence automatically entails via political-aesthetic demarcations. If othering through media presence serves to establish differences as boundaries (between selves and within the self itself) and thus constitutes social structures as power hierarchies, our argument is that compresence establishes connecting relations. In compresence, entities are together for a social and shared, non-segregating reason, which means that one's presence can only be understood in the social, relational sense of a shared presence. This implies care and concern for each other. Compresence is a shared presence, whereas copresent entities are completely independent of each other although they gather in the same space.

Thus, the prefix "com" in com-presence stands for: community, commonality, communication. But it also stands for the mediality of the common, i.e. for computation and, in times of the platform economy, also for commercialization and commodification. In philosophy, the concept of compresence is usually used for ontological and phenomenological argumentation. While we do not intend to reproduce this philosophical discourse and its subtleties in detail here, we would still like to outline the following four common features of its use to underpin our understanding of the term: First, as differently as the concept is interpreted by Plato (2007), Gottfried-Wilhelm Leibniz (2002), Edmund Husserl (1973 and 1976), in bundle theory or in tropical ontology (Denkel 1997; Trettin 2000 and 2001), it refers to special, singular qualities of an entity.

These qualities cannot be essentialized or universalized, but they result from the differences and similarities between the individuals in whom the qualities materialize. Second, this means that qualities are always to be understood as individual, not as universal properties, and thus occur only in relation to other qualities. The qualities are variably and dependently compresent;[5] they exist in an ontological dependence. Third, the term is often used to explain how individuals are constituted—including the difference between the self and the Other, as we noted in the case of othering. In some, though not all, philosophical contexts, for example in Husserl's work (1973 and 1977), compresence does involve a difference between one's own, the inner, and the other, the perception of the outer, but only in order to think about the difference as a common, non-competing compresence. This experience of the unity of what is outwardly physical and what is inwardly felt constitutes the individual. Fourth, all theories of compresence have in common that they are committed to realism, not idealism. The relational and differentiated qualities have their own reality beyond the categories of description and cognition.

This idea of a presentative 'being related to each other,' which also concerns self-perception and the perception of others, can now be linked to medial factors in order to clarify why compresence adequately describes a solidary, social togetherness in the form of medial presence. The ambivalence of presence is revealed in co- and compresence as a negotiation, dynamization, and multiplication of binary structures such as proximity and distance, self and Other, on-screen and off-screen, real and virtual.[6] In what follows, we want to explore what we mean by compresence with regard to what Jan Distelmeyer calls a "symptomatic experiential space" (2021; translated by Elisa Linseisen) of the COVID-19 pandemic and thus also of media presence: the Zoom room.

## Co(m)presence in the Zoom Room

Most of the popular videoconferencing tools that gained widespread usage during the pandemic (Zoom, Skype, Teams, Jitsi, Big Blue Button, etc.) share

---

5    An exception to this is Leibniz (2002), for whom compresence means the copresence of two entities (monads) that are to be regarded as completely separate, holistic, and independent.

6    The negotiation of this ambivalence found expression during the pandemic, for example, in the hashtag #TogetherApart (see e.g. Anderson and kumar Putta 2021).

the same structure and aesthetics: They offer a window which (besides a small toolbar, a chat and participants list) is mainly filled with smaller windows (also called "tiles" or "squares") that represent the members of the meeting—either by showing them via video thumbnail[7] (when their camera is on) or as a black square with only a name on it (when their camera is off or they do not have one). This grid aesthetic thus promises options of virtual copresence and participation—which is what companies like Zoom state in their advertisements; but reality nevertheless showed that these virtual rooms were not made for everyone as they reproduced cultural and societal forms of inequality and exclusion (e.g. in terms of accessibility of technical equipment and broadband internet or the visibility of the private in public, cf. Bautista 2020; Keidl et al. 2020; Katz et al. 2021; Nunes and Ozog 2021). Moreover, the widespread use of videoconferencing tools produced new forms of mental overload and thus inattentiveness/mental absence ("zoom fatigue") (Lovink 2020), and involved ecopolitical dimensions regarding climate change awareness (e.g. in terms of saving electricity by switching off the camera) (Obringer et al. 2021; Travers 2021).

Additionally, as mentioned above, Zoom fostered processes of self-othering, which Zimmermann describes as a result of gaze relations:

> Am I a virtual me or a virtual you? If the person I see on screen is me, it is suggested that it is me who looks at an image of myself on screen. I am the subject that looks at me—and at others. If the person I see on screen is you, the perspective changes. For this suggests that it is the others who look at an image of myself on screen. I am the object of their look—while I am at the same time the object of my look. Ultimately, I am both subject and object of my look. I see myself at once as self and other, as one self/other among others, a split perception of self/other on a splitscreen. (Zimmermann 2020, 100)

Besides the focus on the 'self and/as other,' what becomes apparent in Zimmermann's description is that it is not only the 'self' and the 'others' that are involved in this interplay of gazes; it is the technology as well that 'sees' and 'is

---

7    The arrangement of the thumbnails can be adjusted and ordered according to different types of hierarchy, though—e.g. when you change from "gallery mode" to "speaker mode" thus only enhancing the speaking person's tile while others are moved to the side, or when you 'pin' single thumbnails to keep them present all the time while others might disappear from your view.

seen.' Zoom-users do not look at each other, first of all, they look at a screen. Geert Lovink therefore describes the videoconference setting as a mélange of self, others, and media that inevitably contains a political dimension and thus forms—with reference to Søren Pold—a "Zoomopticon," which he defines as "the condition in which you cannot see if somebody or something is watching you, but it might be the case that you're being watched by both people and corporate software" (2020, 14). What is described here are therefore various forms of othering that occur between selves and media and that are strongly linked to questions of presence. From a media studies perspective, this media involvement is central: Videoconferencing produces different Others regarding technological, mental, physical, and temporal accessibility as well as self-perception. Even more importantly, it is a setting in which hardware and software medially process these types of othering into an audiovisual arrangement of presence on the screen and in the speakers. In short: Zoom turns presence into an aesthetic form.

Critics of Zoom tend to perceive the tool as a technological setting that aims to substitute physical copresence, instead of understanding it as an audiovisual interface that facilitates compresence. What do we mean by that? Distelmeyer, for example, describes the usage of Zoom as a disappointment and an endeavor that, even though it is "beautiful," is painful due to its substitutive function: "The desperate attempt to transfer established and familiar forms of communities 'directly' into internet relationships always also recalls what is missing. To this day, it provokes the beautiful phantom pains of a presence with all those others who must never have been merely dear to us, only to miss them now nonetheless" (2021; translated by Julia Eckel). Following statements like these, it is a diminished, insufficient effect of presence that we experience in Zoom, because we compare it to (a spatiotemporally shared face-to-face) copresence. This disappointment is most pronounced when the audiovisual performance lags behind, which—again—turns non-copresence into an aesthetic effect when faces are glitching and frozen, voices muted or sped up. But still, the arrangement of the tiles, the presence of names and/or faces and voices suggests a certain 'togetherness' as an aesthetic effect. This is not an equalizing presence of 'we are all the same' and 'everything is as usual' (which means outside of the Zoom room without a pandemic going on), but a compresence of individuals that points to and accepts differences without othering them. Hence, the Zoom room interface can also be read and used as a surface that documents who is missing from a meeting or course, who wants to be seen or heard und who cannot or does not want to be seen or heard. So while mourning the inevitable lack of copresence that the tedious and tiring usage of the software during the pandemic has definitely proven, we propose a complementing shift of focus towards compresence. Thus, we seek to offer a term and theoretical concept that allows to describe the Zoom experience of presence more thoroughly—without just saying, that it is not the same as copresence, but by stating: it is also a form of audiovisual compresence, with all its potentials.

## Audiovisual Compresence as Filmic Trans/Individuation

To describe this type of compresence in a bit more detail, let us take a little detour to pre-pandemic times when videoconferencing was not an everyday habit and fate of the masses. A film studies perspective allows us to identify specific aesthetic indicators of audiovisual compresence. Following Julia Bee's (2019) approach on *cinematic trans/individuation* and her feminist reading of the film *Long Story Short* (2016), by director Natalie Bookchin, various aesthetic elements—like split screens and gazes—can be identified as possibilities for collectivization, solidarization, and, hence, compresence.

The stylistic appearance of *Long Story Short* resembles the now familiar surface of Zoom. Thus, the US documentary is an example of a pre-pandemic audiovisual arrangement that demonstrates the aesthetic-political potential of compresence.[8] The film features various interview scenes with people experiencing homelessness in the Bay Area of California and montages the frames and the people appearing and speaking in them against a black background in the tiled look that became ubiquitous in videoconferencing during the pandemic (fig. 6 and 7). As Bee points out, this "formal design makes it possible, through the talking heads arranged in the split screen, to create a public sphere that negotiates a problem coextensive with feminism: the politicization of the personal as a negotiation of difference, and thus the question of the agency of the collective that emerges from and constitutes it" (2019, 4–5; translated by Elisa Linseisen). In the film, three axes of relations are established that create compresence and therefore might be transferable to Zoom: first, the compresence between the people in the pictorial, audiovisual space. Their relationship is created by the split screens, the montage of images and sound—the voices that circulate across the frame (fig. 6). Bookchin conducted the interviews

---

8    The trailer and a short excerpt of the film can be seen online (Bookchin 2016b and 2016c; last accessed June 8, 2023).

completely independently. The arrangement of people sitting calmly, looking intently into the camera, gives the impression that they are present together, listening to each other and sometimes speaking together. Bookchin assembles the statements of the interviewees like a chorus, generating a collective voice that is not merely reactive, but fluid between the split screens (fig. 7). The film creates an aesthetic that never gives the impression of a holistic unity. Rather, a representative collective emerges in the difference. It is the presence of difference of the interviewees in the medial, in the pictorial space, and the camera's view of this space that creates a community.

The second compresent relationship emerges between the people in the image and the viewers. Through the arrangement that resembles that of a video conference, the statements of the collective of people appear to be addressed to each other on the one hand, and to the audience on the other (fig. 7). Even if it is not a matter of presuming to belong to a collective that shares its quite painful experiences through copresence, a commonality of social responsibility is created by looking into the camera. According to our approach, this can be distinguished from othering, also because the spectator's own presence, which does not appear on the screen (after all, it is still a film and not a video conference), has no self-reflexive dimensions. The spectator's presence lies in being addressed, in listening and in (silent) participation—a presence that corresponds to many moments in Zoom spaces, especially when taking part with your camera off.

The third relationship is that between those present and their mediatization, which is consolidated in the (split) screen as well as in front of the screen in the role of purely audiovisual individuals (or in short: audioviduals; see Eckel 2021). All the people in the picture, the interviewer, and the audience are connected by the aesthetic form of a medial presence. Even if the audience does not 'really' interact with the persons, a form of presence and a culture of affect and social participation is established through the film-aesthetic arrangement, the 'bringing together' of voices, faces, and backgrounds and the stories they share. The screen gathers these individuals on the same level/medial surface but nevertheless accepts, supports, even depends on their individuality and differences.

*Figures 6 & 7: Filmic arrangement of split screens and gazes. Screenshots taken from* Long Story Short *(2016).*

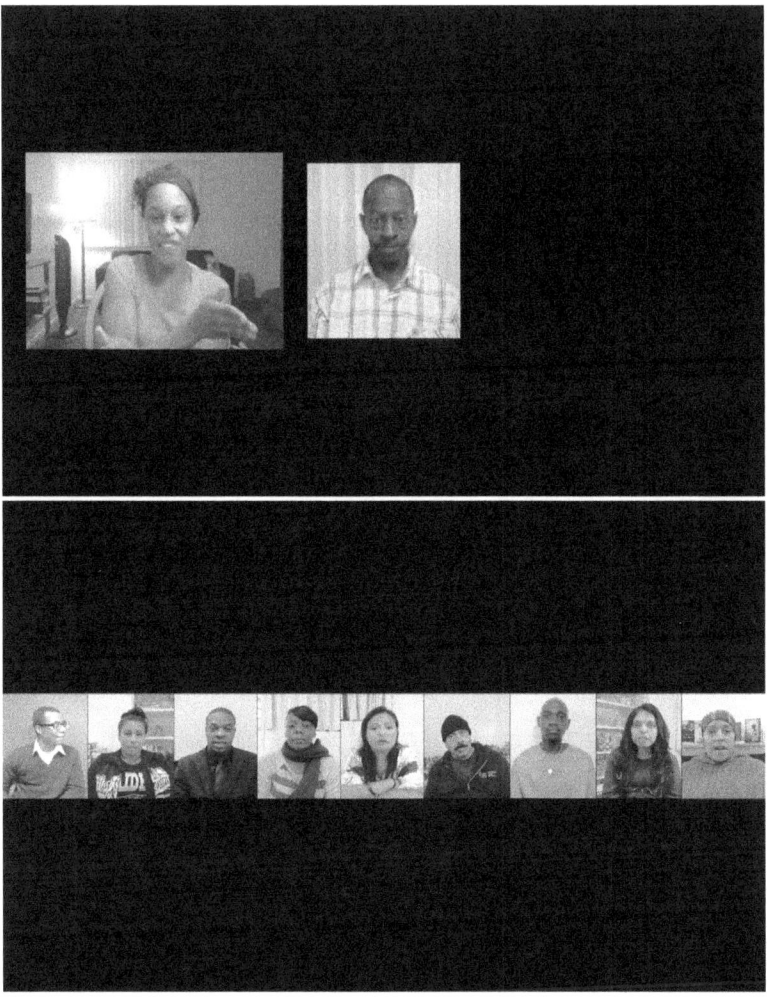

What the moving image and its aesthetic potentials (split screens, gazes into the camera, montaging of people, things, words, sounds, etc.) offer is therefore an audiovisually perceptible 'commonality of individuality' that Bee describes (in reference to Gilbert Simondon's concept of individuation) as a *cinematic trans/individuation*. According to this idea, film is considered as a (potentially) "performative, actualizing, and expressive act that does not show what already exists (one identity and then a second, for comparison), but rather takes seriously the mediality of this endeavor: a *cinematic* trans/individuation that lies in exploring the potential of film to produce publics" (Bee 2019, 10; translated by Julia Eckel).[9] Cinematic trans/individuation can therefore be understood as an aesthetic way of creating compresence on a screen, a process that is transferable to the Zoom room as an aesthetical, audiovisual, moving image interface as well.

## Share the Square

In the following, we will transfer these ideas to the Zoom setting and identify components that facilitate a similar kind of aesthetic trans/individuation and thus audiovisual compresence. For us, there seem to be three aspects that are relevant in this regard: compresence with 'others,' compresence with environments, and compresence with media.

---

9    Bee refers to Muriel Combes here who describes Simondon's idea of individuation as transferable to groups as well: "[A] Group for Simondon is not a simple assemblage of individuals, but the very movement of self-constitution of the collective .... Such an individuation is at once an individuation of *the group* and an individuation of *grouped individuals*, which are inseparable." (Combes 2013, 43).

## Compresence with Others—Talking Heads and Split Screens

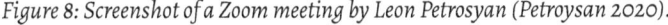

*Figure 8: Screenshot of a Zoom meeting by Leon Petrosyan (Petroysan 2020).*

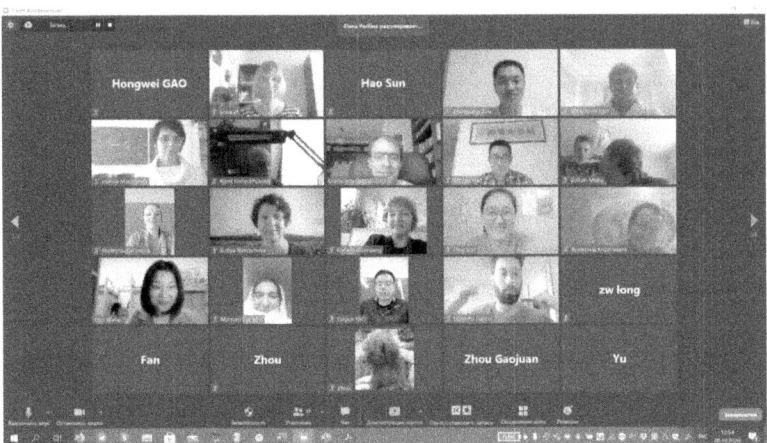

The split screen[10] aesthetics of Zoom and the frontal gaze into the camera are the most obvious parallel between the film analyzed above and the Zoom interface. Thus, the whole design of Zoom serves the purpose of building types of on-screen-communities—which is doomed to disappoint as long as these are interpreted as a gathering of medially equalized and at the same time othered individuals instead of a process of medially performed individuation. Additionally, it is important to understand the shift of focus of our argumentation compared to the Zoom-critical voices cited above: Of course, the grid pattern of Zoom, the dark lines that separate the tiles, can be read as a barrier between people, as a separation that medially points to their non-co-presence and otherness (not only regarding the fact that they are not present in a room with you and medially transformed but referring to structures of social and political othering as well). However, at the same time the 'gallery view' creates its own kind of media-aesthetic togetherness that results from the arrangement of the split screen and the affective gaze structure established as a webcam-induced norm. And even if the camera is switched off, the compresence of the 'black tile' and (usually) a name testifies that someone has at least

---

10    For a short overview on the history of the split screen in its relation to Zoom, see Hagener 2020.

entered the meeting and thus considers their virtual presence (without being seen and maybe even heard) useful or necessary. Hence, the tile represents an idea of presence; even if the person behind it should be factually absent, their visual 'rectangular substitute' becomes part of the aesthetic screen ornament of Zoom.

What Zoom's design offers is therefore maybe comparable to forms of social media protest and hashtag-activism that often start with building a shared tile-aesthetic, for example, the many black thumbnails on Instagram as a sign of solidarity with 'Blackout Tuesday' and the BlackLivesMatter movement (Uca 2021; Wellman 2022)[11] or social media selfie-campaigns like #BlackOutDay or #transdayofvisibility where Black and trans* people shared selfies to reach a higher representation on Twitter, Facebook, and other platforms with the aim to deconstruct stereotypes (Tan 2015; Thomas 2015; Strudwick 2015). Even though the 'only images' might refer to a physical absence of the people (compared to a street protest, for example),[12] they nevertheless open new rooms to act and to build an alternative, additional, or integral type of community—constructed out of individuals that share (image) actions and aesthetics. The Zoom interface can therefore be read as a shared space to be designed by its users as well (even if it is only within the narrow options that the software supplies). Leaving the camera off, then, becomes an aesthetic and political statement or even just an individual choice that nevertheless points to the politics of Zoom via an aesthetic decision (to become a black tile in

11    This campaign is very interesting regarding the logics of online protest via social media and the question of allyship because it did not work out as the initiators intended. Planned as a campaign to reflect on the huge impact of Black music and artists in the music industry and as a sign for solidarity with the BlackLivesMatter movement by artists from the Black community, the habit to post a black square on your Instagram account has soon be appropriated by *white* users as well and by people who did not know about the initial cause (the BlackoutTuesday campaign) because they thought it was 'only' a trending sign for solidarity with BlackLivesMatter (which led to criticism by BLM activists). Here again, we thus find a striking example for an aesthetic form of visual/medial compresence (the grid of black tiles as a sign for solidarity with Black music culture and anti-racism, but at the same time the politics of this setting as the people/users 'behind' the squares were in some cases not intended to take part). Who and what is present on the screen and who is represented thereby become important questions that can be described with ideas of copresence and compresence.

12    Some forms of social media protest and solidarity declarations are therefore often criticized as slacktivism, a term which blames these types of actions to be only a minimal effort that does not help to achieve larger political goals (Dennis 2019, 6–7).

the gallery). Read this way, the software produces its own kinds of presences which result from the aesthetic copresence of squares that are interpreted as a compresence of their users.

## Compresence with the Environment—Bodies and Backgrounds

The relevance of the square design in Zoom applies not only to the subject in its center, but also to its surrounding. Thus, in the course of the pandemic, lively debates emerged about the importance of backgrounds in videoconferencing situations. These debates gained special prominence through the Twitter account Room Rater that started in April 2020 with the mission to evaluate image backgrounds of video call guests (usually on TV) with a 10-point scheme and to create a kind of catalog of successful Zoom-oriented room designs. The account-owners eventually compiled their findings in a book called *How to Zoom Your Room: Room Rater's Ultimate Style Guide* (Taylor and Bahrey 2022) which includes tips on the best arrangement of bookshelves, the relevance of plants in the picture, the choice of furniture and wall decor, and no-go's of videoconferencing such as the "hostage video situation" (6) (fig. 9).

The Room Rater project serves as another example for our argument regarding the ambivalent relation of pandemic othering and compresence. The book starts by describing the potential of public video calls precisely as a counter-mechanism to the effects of othering occurring in both pandemic and pre-pandemic times:

> The virus exposed inequalities and deep divisions in society, but one democratizing effect was that we got a chance to see how our favorite journalists, political pundits, and celebrities lived when not in a studio. We saw the art, décor and 'stuff,' but also the messy rooms, rambunctious children, and photo-bombing pets. It was in this climate that Room Rater struck a collective nerve. (Taylor and Bahrey 2022, 3)

*Figure 9: Ideal Zoom-backgrounds in* How to Zoom Your Room: Room Rater's Ultimate Style Guide *(Taylor and Bahrey 2022, i).*

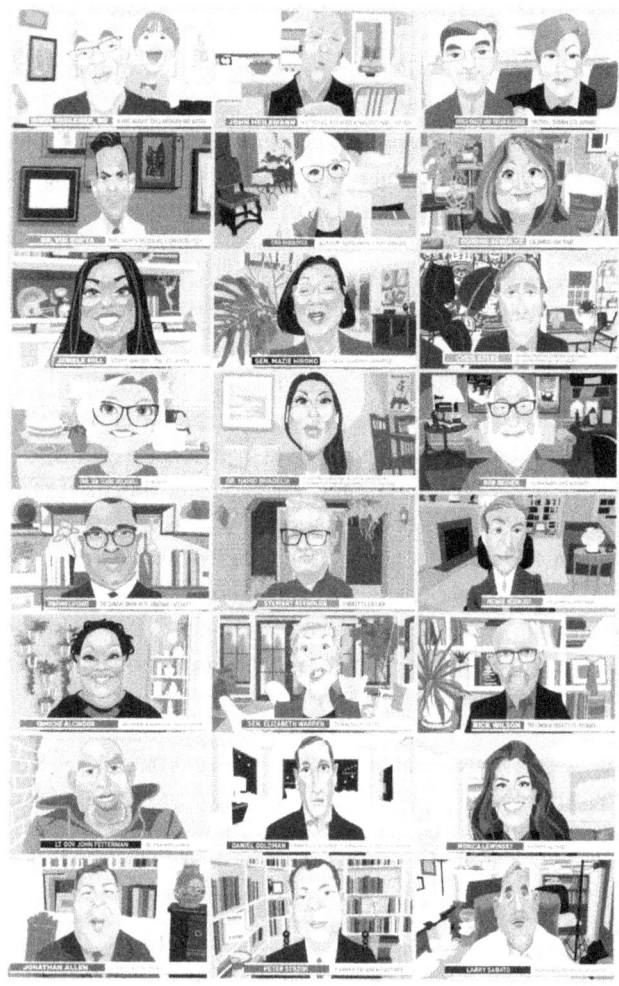

The democratizing effects of Zoom—according to this argumentation—therefore emerged from the equalizing force to stay at home and to publicly disclose this private space as part of working in home office. As this force applied to 'regular workers'[13] as well as to public figures, who usually only appeared in professional settings and sets before, videoconferencing thus seemingly crossed class and power hierarchies by showing that the privileged ones are 'only people at home' as well. The discussion of their interiors and living spaces—as carried out by the Room Rater account—hence enabled a feeling of rapprochement ('we're all the same in a videocall square') and at the same time, through evaluation and ranking, even a form of reciprocal empowerment that was able to counter the inequality and the othering between 'us down here' and 'them up there'—at least, that is the interpretation of the book. This reading, of course, does not take into account that the othering between 'those public figures on TV' (that are worth rating) and those Others in private spaces persists, not to mention the ones who are not able to work from home, not equipped to be present in a Zoom call, or ashamed to disclose the place they are in.

The book nevertheless holds on to the dehierarchizing effects of its How-to-advice by stating that the "style guide is for everyone," that it offers "simple, inexpensive, and easily achieved" solutions and that it needs only "a little bit of effort and savvy" and small "additions such as plants, pets, and even an appearance by a child or two" that are able to create "warmth and a sense of camaraderie to any sterile conference call" (Taylor and Bahrey 2022, 6). The "camaraderie" of Zoom is revealed here as a superficial show effect that does not have to have anything to do with your real life or your actual surrounding—as long as the square complies to the Room Rater standards (with pets and children added to the field of interior design). The idea of 'real' representation and copresence is therefore dismissed in favor of a universal design concept that manages to equalize a society by just hiding or enhancing what is 'real' beyond the mise-en-scène of the Zoom frame. The background design is presented as an answer to class inequalities, but is in fact subjected to a thoroughly neoliberal logic of self-optimization (as spatial optimization). Even if Room Rater only seems to rearrange the othering (the Others are the ones with the bad zoom backgrounds now), social othering remains something that has to be concealed, according to this logic.

---

13    The book's argument falls a bit short in this regard, of course, because it does not consider the fact that being able to work from home is itself in many cases a cause of privilege and thus produces forms of othering: between people who are forced to leave their home for (often physical and in many cases less paid) work while home office is an option for people doing (often better paid) mental and conceptual work.

Despite all these critical aspects that might come up in the reading of the book, there is still a dimension of compresence that the Room Rater example points to—the relation between individual and background in Zoom. Besides the intentionally anthropocentric arrangement of videoconferencing, the (talking) heads and bodies within the frames merge with their environment on the surface of the screen—be it a study, kitchen, bedroom or a white wall, a blurry surface or an artificially inserted background with glitches between body and surrounding. Hence, the othering between non-living and living, human and non-human appears leveled through the aesthetic arrangement, especially because of the strong link of the subject to 'home' and 'office' as two important spaces of self-definition (at least in modern capitalism). Understood this way, Zoom creates a visual symbiosis between individual and environment and—beyond all critique—offers a scope to explore and negotiate this demarcation.

The deconstructive dimension and the challenging of established differentiations like subject/object, living/thing, nature/culture therefore invokes a potentiality of "otherness" (Haraway 2003) as proposed by post-humanist or new materialist approaches (e.g. Barad 2007). It is the compresence with our environments—what Haraway terms "significant otherness" or "otherness-in-connection" (2003, 45), meaning "patterns within which the players are neither wholes nor parts" (8) – that is displayed in the Zoom square(s). These at the same time aesthetic, technological, and social features of Zoom have the potential to counteract the othering of copresence.

## Compresence with Media—Monitoring Monitors

A third dimension of compresence focuses on the even wider frame of Zoom. The fact that Zoom users do not look at 'oneself' and 'others' but at a screen has gained a certain prominence during the pandemic, because suddenly the copresence with screens became more visible—e.g. when thinking about the presence of monitors as a substitute for guests in TV studio settings (fig. 10). To show screens on screen in a kind of self-reflexive metalepsis therefore emerged as a standard element of broadcasting; it turned our view of screens into a "screen image" (Gerling, Möring, and De Mutiis 2023) which put our copresence with screens itself on view. At the same time, the setting presented the absence of, for example, talkshow guests, 're-presentified' by monitor versions of them, as a sufficient substitute that pretended not to turn them into mediated Others but equal participants of the discussion (fig. 10). These diegetic split screens therefore generate an effect of compresence that points to our entanglement with technology.

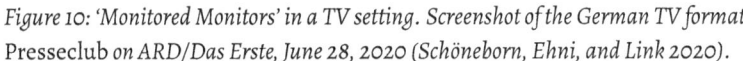

*Figure 10: 'Monitored Monitors' in a TV setting. Screenshot of the German TV format* Presseclub *on ARD/Das Erste, June 28, 2020 (Schöneborn, Ehni, and Link 2020).*

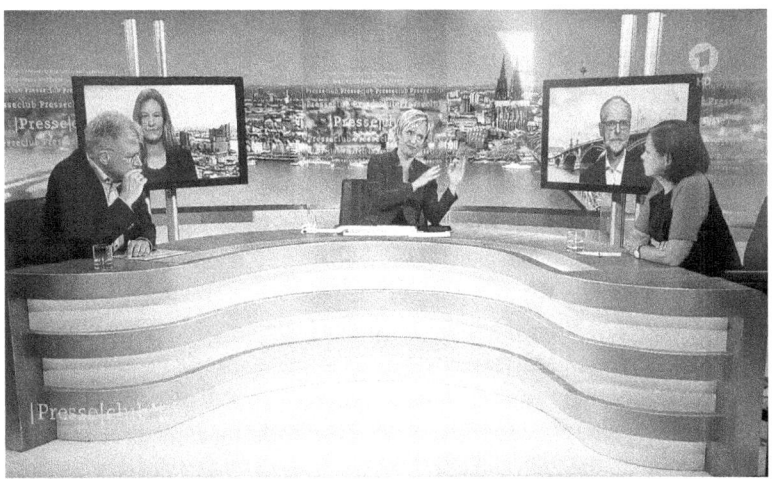

During the COVID-19 pandemic and particularly through quarantine, the interfaces of laptops, tablets, TVs, and mobile media technologies evolved into windows to the world and 'gatekeepers' that channeled the knowledge about the virus and thus defined what was experienced as the 'pandemic condition' in the first place. While being informed about the global scope of the virus outbreak as a worldwide issue, the screens concomitantly delimited an intimate field which separated the public from the subjective sphere. Screens thus allowed us to keep distance through them, just to find presence on them.

This copresence with media technologies—and especially screens—therefore is an aspect that is strongly connected to videoconferencing software like Zoom. The monitoring of our encounters with monitors even got implemented into the Zoom experience itself because the software allows to record its meetings with its build-in-recording function.[14] The screen and its (in most cases

---

14    What happens here is a form of screencasting that always implies a certain self-reflexivity of media (see e.g. Eckel (2023) for a short history of screencasting or Distelmeyer (2023) on the genre of desktop movies as a related phenomenon).

frame-integrated) webcam therefore became an instrument of participation as well as of documentation and surveillance. It allowed to watch and film people interacting with screens (which themselves show people interacting with screens) on screen and to reproduce this on screen – without even showing one of these screens directly. What a complex entanglement.

Being informed by the software about the recording (via voice and text message and through a red record-button in the corner) turns the presentation of your individual face and body, surrounded by your home/office or other environments, into something that is othered through the recording, because this arrangement is not only disclosed to the people that are in the meeting with you but potentially shared independently of you and the Zoom room within other contexts.

This type of 'othering' (that gives others and the software the opportunity to share your presence independently of you) again points towards forms of compresence as well. The recordings of our copresence with screen media—be it in a TV studio setting or within a recorded Zoom meeting—invoke general ideas of a compresence with technology as the boundaries between me in front of the screen, me (and my background) on the screen, and the screen itself are blurred. There is no divide between 'me here' and 'the medium there' as something other(ed); the individuation happens in-between, in the processuality and referenciality of the encounter. The fact that screens and the people using them are filmed therefore points to a further dimension of filmic trans/individuation connected to an aesthetic experience of compresence surrounding Zoom.

In total, the square of Zoom is therefore shared not only with yourself and others but also with your environment and the medial setting it involves. It may serve as a medial framing of a copresence of othered individuals, but also as a medium of an aesthetically perceivable trans/individuating compresence in which self, other, and medium constitute themselves dependently.[15]

## Conclusion

The argument unfolded here can be summarized as follows: In order to understand the effects and affects that Zoom produces with respect to individuals and society, the medial surface of this software must be taken into ac-

---

15    This paragraph summarizes the findings of the last three subchapters.

count as an aesthetic form. Our proposal has been to examine Zoom in terms of presence effects, which are characterized by two tendencies—copresence and compresence. The problem of the lack of spatiotemporal, mostly physically conceived copresence is one of the major criticisms of the use of Zoom, combined with further related othering effects that (re)produce political and social inequalities. These points have been intensively addressed and discussed by critics in the debate about videoconferencing during the pandemic. Neglected, however, have been the 'compresential' aspects of Zoom which emerge primarily from its purely medial, audiovisual surface and are to be analyzed as an aesthetic presence effect. This is not intended to establish a counter position to the justified criticism of the disadvantages, shortcomings, and inadequacies of videoconferencing or a relativization of its othering and discriminating effects, but on the contrary as a complementary focus on the aesthetic surface of the tools and software used as a medial structure for audiovisual gatherings. Taking a closer look at these aesthetic aspects promises to provide important impulses for working with software like Zoom, because in many contexts videoconferencing will certainly stay present even in post-pandemic times. A focus on the 'copresentative' as well as 'compresentative' aspects can therefore help us to use the software in awareness of its othering effects and the flaws of non-copresence, while also searching for potentials of togetherness and community building in its usage as well. [16] To understand Zoom as an amalgam of technological, societal, and aesthetic aspects means to see the Zoom screen as an ornament of faces, forms, and backgrounds, as a shared and collectively formable square.

## Works Cited

Anderson, Bissie, and Santhosh kumar Putta. 2021. "Introduction: #TogetherApart: Mediatization, (Inter)subjectivity and Sociality at a Time of Pan-

---

16    For two creative examples that use the interface aesthetics of videoconferencing tools as a basis for a collaborative artwork see the music videos 日々の音色 *(Hibi no neiro)* by SOUR (masakaa 2009) and *Phenom* by Thao and the Get Down Stay Down (2020). Both use the tile aesthetics of software like Zoom to create screen ornaments and coordinated performances that connect and overcome the borders of the individual frames presented on screen.

demic." *Networking Knowledge: Journal of the MeCCSA Postgraduate Network* 14, no. 1: 1–8. https://doi.org/10.31165/nk.2021.141.663.

Ashcroft, Bill, Gareth Griffiths, and Helen Tiffin. 2007. *Post-Colonial Studies: The Key Concepts*. 2nd Edition. London: Routledge.

Barad, Karen. 2007. *Meeting the Universe Halfway: Quantum Physics and the Entanglement of Matter and Meaning*. Durham: Duke University Press.

Bautista, Nidia. 2020. "Distance Learning During Coronavirus Worsens Race, Class Inequality in Education." *Teen Vogue*. May 1, 2020. https://www.teen vogue.com/story/distance-learning-low-income-students.

Bee, Julia. 2019. "Filmische Trans/Individuationen. Ansprache, Affekte und die Konstitution von feministischen Kollektiven in LONG STORY SHORT und YOURS IN SISTERHOOD." *Nachdemfilm No. 17: Feminismus und Film*. https://nachdemfilm.de/issues/text/filmische-transindividuationen.

Benjamin, Walter. (1935) 2013. *Das Kunstwerk im Zeitalter seiner technischen Reproduzierbarkeit: Werke und Nachlass. Kritische Gesamtausgabe*. Vol. 16. Edited by Burkhardt Lindner, Simon Broll, and Jessica Nitsche. Berlin: Suhrkamp.

Bergermann, Ulrike, and Nanna Heidenreich. 2015. *total.—Universalismus und Partikularismus in post_kolonialer Medientheorie*. Bielefeld: transcript.

Bookchin, Natalie, dir. 2016a. *Long Story Short*. USA, Icarus Films. Dafilms, https://dafilms.com/film/9911-long-story-short?rc=US.

———, dir. 2016b. *Long Story Short: Trailer*. https://longstory.us.

———, dir. 2016c. *Long Story Short: Excerpt*. https://bookchin.net/projects/long -story-short/.

Bowyer, Dorothea, Milissa Deitz, Anne Jamison, Chloe E. Taylor, Erika Gyengesi, Jaime Ross, Hollie Hammond, Anita Eseosa Ogbeide, and Tinashe Dune. 2021. "Academic Mothers, Professional Identity and COVID-19: Feminist Reflections on Career Cycles, Progression and Practice." *Gender, Work & Organization* 29, no. 1: 309–41. https://doi.org/10.1111/gwao.12750.

Bracken, Cheryl Campanella. 2005. "Presence and Image Quality: The Case of High-Definition Television." *Media Psychology*, no. 7: 191–205. https://www.tandfonline.com/doi/abs/10.1207/S1532785XMEP0702_4.

Cefai, Sarah, and Nick Couldry. 2019. "Mediating the Presence of Others: Reconceptualising Co-Presence as Mediated Intimacy." *European Journal of Cultural Studies* 22, no. 3: 291–308. https://doi.org/10.1177/1367549417743040.

Combes, Muriel. 2013. *Gilbert Simondon and the Philosophy of the Transindividual*. Translated by Thomas LaMarre. London: MIT Press.

"Compresence." n.d. *Merriam-Webster Dictionary*. Last Accessed June 22, 2023. https://www.merriam-webster.com/dictionary/compresence.

"Copresence." n.d. *Merriam-Webster Dictionary*. Last Accessed June 22, 2023. https://www.merriam-webster.com/dictionary/copresence.

Denkel, Arda. 1997. "On the Compresence of Tropes." *Philosophy and Phenomenological Research* 57, no. 3 (September): 599–606. https://doi.org/10.2307/2953751.

Dennis, James. 2019. *Beyond Slacktivism: Political Participation on Social Media*. Cham: Springer Nature/Palgrave Macmillan.

De Rosa, Anamaria Silvana, and Terri Mannarini. 2021. "Covid-19 as an 'Invisible Other' and Socio-Spatial Distancing Within a One-Metre Individual Bubble." *Urban Design International* 26: 370–90. https://doi.org/10.1057/s41289-021-00151-z.

Derrida, Jaques. 2003. *Eine gewisse unmögliche Möglichkeit, vom Ereignis zu sprechen*. Translated by Susanne Lüdemann. Berlin: Merve.

Distelmeyer, Jan. 2021. "Programmatische Verhältnisse. Wer oder was lebt in Zoom? Fragen an die neue Normalität von Videokonferenzen." *CARGO* 49 (March): 28–34.

———. 2023. "A Case for Interface Studies: From Screenshots to Desktop/Screen Films." In *Screen Images: Screenshot, Screencast, In-Game Photography*, edited by Winfried Gerling, Sebastian Möring, and Marco De Mutiis, 317–32. Berlin: Kadmos. https://doi.org/10.55309/c3ie61k5.

Dudley, Daria. 2022. "'Systemic Relevance' for Social Work: More than Just a Compliment—Not Yet a Proper Law. An Evaluation of Pandemic-Related Legal Changes in Germany." In *Covid, Crisis, Care, and Change? International Gender Perspectives on Re/Production, State and Feminist Transitions*, edited by Antonia Kupfer and Constanze Stutz, 59–72. Opladen: Verlag Barbara Budrich. https://doi.org/10.3224/84742541.

Eckel, Julia. 2021. *Das Audioviduum. Eine Theoriegeschichte des Menschenmotivs in audiovisuellen Medien*. Bielefeld: transcript.

———. 2023. "Screencasting: Documenting Processuality." In *Screen Images: Screenshot, Screencast, In-Game Photography*, edited by Winfried Gerling, Sebastian Möring, and Marco De Mutiis, 341–70. Berlin: Kadmos. https://doi.org/10.55309/c3ie61k5.

Eickelmann, Jennifer, Sophie G. Einwächter, Felix Gregor, Ulrike Hanstein, Sandra Kero, and Elisa Linseisen. 2021. *Handreichung zur Gewaltprävention in Lehr- und Lernkontexten online. media/rep/*. https://doi.org/10.25969/mediarep/15780.

Ernst, Christoph, and Heike Paul, eds. 2013. *Präsenz und Implizites Wissen*. Bielefeld: transcript.

Fernández, María. 1999. "Postcolonial Media Theory." *Art Journal* 58, no. 3 (Autumn): 58–73. http://www.jstor.org/stable/777861?origin=JSTOR-pdf.

Foster, Thomas. 1997. "'Trapped by the Body?' Telepresence Technologies and Transgendered Performance in Feminist and Lesbian Rewritings of Cyperpunk Fiction." *Modern Fiction Studies* 43, no. 3, (Fall): 708–742. http://www.jstor.org/stable/26285657.

França, Thais. 2022. "'No Less of a Woman': Examining the (Invisible) Life of Childfree Women Academics during the COVID-19 Pandemic." *Journal of Gender Studies* 31, no. 8: 956–68. https://doi.org/10.1080/09589236.2022.2125863.

Gerling, Winfried, Sebastian Möring, and Marco de Mutiis, Marco, eds. *Screen-Images: Screenshot, Screencast, In-Game Photography*. Berlin: Kadmos. https://doi.org/10.55309/c3ie61k5.

Gumbrecht, Hans Ulrich. 2003. *Production of Presence: What Meaning Cannot Convey*. Stanford: Stanford University Press.

———. 2014. *Our Broad Present: Time and Contemporary Culture*. New York: Columbia University Press.

Haden, Heather Jean. 2015. *The Aesthetics of Unease: Telepresence Art and Hyper-Subjectivity*. M.A. thesis. College of the Arts, Kent State University. https://etd.ohiolink.edu/apexprod/rws_etd/send_file/send?accession=kent1429862881&disposition=inline.

Hagener, Malte. 2020. "Divided, Together, Apart: How Split Screen Became Our Everyday Reality." In *Pandemic Media: Preliminary Notes Toward an Inventory*, edited by Philipp Dominik Keidl, Laliv Melamed, Vinzenz Hediger, and Antonio Somaini, 33–42. Bielefeld: transcript.

Haraway, Donna. 2003. *The Companion Species Manifestó: Dogs, People, and Significant Otherness*. Chicago: Prickly Paradigm Press.

Husserl, Edmund. 1973. *Gesammelte Werke: Band XV/3. Zur Phänomenologie der Intersubjektivität. Dritter Teil: 1929–1935*. Edited by Iso Kern. Den Haag: Martinus Nijhoff.

———. 1976. *Gesammelte Werke: Band III/1. Ideen zu einer reinen Phänomenologie und phänomenologische Philosophie. Erstes Buch: Allgemeine Einführung in die reine Phänomenologie*. Edited by Karl Schuhmann. Den Haag: Martinus Nijhoff.

Katz, Vikki S., Amy B. Jordan, and Katherine Ognyanova. 2021. "Digital Inequality, Faculty Communication, and Remote Learning Experiences during the COVID-19 Pandemic: A Survey of U.S. Undergraduates." *Plos One* 16, no. 2 (February). https://doi.org/10.1371/journal.pone.0246641.

Keidl, Philipp Dominik, Laliv Melamed, Vinzenz Hediger, and Antonio Somaini, eds. 2020. *Pandemic Media: Preliminary Notes Toward an Inventory.* Lüneburg: Meson Press. https://doi.org/10.25969/mediarep/17192.

Kiening, Christian, ed. 2007. *Mediale Gegenwärtigkeit.* Vol. 1 of *Medienwandel—Medienwechsel—Medienwissen.* Zürich: Chronos. https://doi.org/10.259 69/mediarep/11742.

Leibniz, Gottfried Wilhelm. 2002. *Monadologie und andere metaphysische Schriften.* Edited and translated by Ulrich Johannes Schneider. Hamburg: Felix Meiner Verlag.

Lovink, Geert. 2020. "The Anatomy of Zoom Fatigue." *Eurozine.* November 2, 2020. https://www.eurozine.com/the-anatomy-of-zoom-fatigue/.

masakaa. 2009. "SOUR '日々の音色 (Hibi no neiro).'" Directed by Masashi Kawamura, Hal Kirkland, Magico Nakamura, and Masayoshi Nakamura, uploaded July 1, 2009. YouTube, https://www.youtube.com/watch?v=WfB lUQguvyw.

McLuhan, Marshall. 2001. *Understanding Media: The Extensions of Man.* Abingdon: Routledge.

Merten, Kai, and Lucia Krämer. 2016. *Postcolonial Studies Meets Media Studies: A Critical Encounter.* Bielefeld: transcript.

Milan, Stefania, Emiliano Treré, and Silvia Masiero, eds. 2021. *COVID-19 from the Margins: Pandemic Invisibilities, Policies and Resistance in the Datafied Society.* Amsterdam: Institute of Network Cultures (Theory on Demand 40). ht tps://doi.org/10.25969/mediarep/19260.

Minsky, Marvin. 1980. "Telepresence." *Omni Magazine* (June): 45–51.

Nunes, Mark, and Cassandra Ozog. 2021. "Your (Internet) Connection Is Unstable." *M/C Journal: Zoom* 24, no. 3. https://doi.org/10.5204/mcj.2813.

Obringer, Rennee, Benjamin Rachunok, Debora Maia-Silva, Maryam Arbabzadeh, Rhoshanak Nateghi, and Kaveh Madani. 2021. "The Overlooked Environmental Footprint of Increasing Internet Use." *Resources, Conservation and Recycling* 167 (April). https://www.sciencedirect.com/scie nce/article/abs/pii/S0921344920307072?via%3Dihub.

Parish, Helen. 2020. "The Absence of Presence and the Presence of Absence: Social Distancing, Sacraments, and the Virtual Religious Community during the COVID-19 Pandemic." *Religions* 11, no. 6: 276. https://doi.org/10.3390/r el11060276.

Petrosyan, Leon. "14th International Conference on Game Theory and Management GTM2020 (October 5–9, 2020, Saint Petersburg State University, Saint Petersburg, Russian Federation)." *Wikimedia Commons.* October 5, 2020. https://commons.wikimedia.org/wiki/File:GTM2020-2.png.

Plato. 2007. *Phaidon.* Translated and edited by Barbara Zehnpfennig. Hamburg: Felix Meiner Verlag.

Preciado, Paul B. 2020. "Learning from the Virus." *Artforum* 58, no. 9 (May–June). https://www.artforum.com/print/202005/paul-b-preciado-8 2823.

Rancière, Jacques. 2004. *The Politics of Aesthetics: The Distribution of the Sensible.* New York: Continuum.

Room Rater (@ratemyskyperoom). 2020. Twitter, Joined April 2020. https://tw itter.com/ratemyskyperoom.

Schöneborn, Jörg, Ellen Ehni, and Susan Link, hosts. 2020 *Presseclub: Das Erste (ARD).* ARD Mediathek. June 28, 2020. https://www1.wdr.de/daserste/pre sseclub/index.html.

Siegert, Bernard. 1993. *Relais: Geschicke der Literatur als Epoche der Post.* Berlin: Brinkmann & Bose.

Spagnolli, Anna, Matthew Lombard, and Luciano Gamberini. 2009. "Mediated Presence: Virtual Reality, Mixed Environments and Social Networks." *Virtual Reality*, no. 13: 137–9. https://doi.org/10.1007/s10055-009-0128-z.

Spivak, Gayatri Chakravorty. 1985. "The Rani of Sirmur: An Essay in Reading the Archives." *History and Theory* 24, no. 3 (October): 247–72. https://doi.org /10.2307/2505169.

Strudwick, Patrick. 2015. "These Trans People Are Taking Selfies to Celebrate Transgender Day of Visibility." *Buzzfeed.* March 31, 2015. https://www.buz zfeed.com/patrickstrudwick/these-trans-people-are-taking-selfies-to-ce lebrate-transgend#.pdx8KvjZP.

Tan, Avianne. 2015. "#BlackOutDay: Trending Twitter Hashtag Celebrates Black People, Fights Negative Stereotypes." *abc News.* March 6, 2015. https: //abcnews.go.com/US/blackoutday-trending-twitter-hashtag-celebrates -black-people-fights/story?id=29439319.

Taylor, Claude, and Jessie Bahrey. 2022. *How to Zoom Your Room: Room Rater's Ultimate Style Guide.* Illustrated by Chris Morris. New York: Voracious.

Thao & The Get Down Stay Down. "Thao & The Get Down Stay Down—Phenom (Official Music Video)." Directed by Erin S. Murray and Jeremy Schaulin-Rioux, produced by Victoria Fayad, uploaded April 3, 2020.YouTube, https ://www.youtube.com/watch?v=DGwQZrDNLO8.

Thomas, Ebony Elizabeth. 2015. "whatwhiteswillneverknow: Official #Black-outday Masterpost." *The Dark Fantastic: Emancipating the Imagination* (blog). March 6, 2015. https://ebonyteach.tumblr.com/post/112888736788/official -blackoutday-masterpost-welcome-this-is.

Travers, Kelley. 2021. "How to Reduce the Environmental Impact of Your Next Virtual Meeting." *MIT News*. March 4, 2021. https://news.mit.edu/2021/ho w-to-reduce-environmental-impact-next-virtual-meeting-0304.

Trettin, Käthe. 2000. "Gibt es überhaupt Frauen? Ein neuer Versuch, Simone de Beauvoirs klassische Frage zu beantworten." *Feministische Studien* 18, no. 1: 111–21. https://doi.org/10.1515/fs-2000-0110.

———. 2001. "Tropen, Sachverhalte und Prozesse: Kategorien für neue Onto-logien." *Polylog: Zeitschrift für interkulturelles Philosophieren: Neue Ontologien*, no. 7: 81–92.

Uca, Didem. 2021. "White Noise and Black Boxes: Social Justice Discourses and Social Media Practices." *Seminar: A Journal of Germanic Studies* 57, no.3 (August): 310–18. https://doi.org/10.3138/seminar.57.3.Forum004.

Virilio, Paul. 1991. *The Aesthetics of Disappearance*. Translated by Phil Beitchman. Los Angeles: Semiotext(e).

Wellman, Mariah L. 2022. "Black Squares for Black Lives? Performative Ally-ship as Credibility Maintenance for Social Media Influencers on Insta-gram." *Social Media + Society* 8, no. 1. https://doi.org/10.1177/205630512210 80473.

Zimmermann, Yvonne. 2020. "Videoconferencing and the Uncanny Encounter with Oneself: Self-Reflexivity as Self-Monitoring 2.0." In *Pandemic Media: Preliminary Notes Toward an Inventory*, edited by Philipp Dominik Keidl, Laliv Melamed, Vinzenz Hediger, and Antonio Somaini, 99–104. Bielefeld: tran-script.

# 10. The Necropolitics of Breathing: On the Scream as Resistance in Contemporary Sound Performances

*Natalie Pielok*

At the end of August 2021, I attended the festival *Acting in Concert*[1] in Witten, Germany. The small-scale festival was a non-commercial project of the association *raum e.v.*, supported by public cultural funding. The entrance to the festival was free and it was announced to be a safe space for women, queer people and Black People of Color (BPoC), and hence framed as being opposed to the exclusionary structures of much of the club and concert culture (Interkultureller Kalender 2022; Acting in Concert 2021a). It was an event that was particularly appealing to me as a queer and post-migrant person, and I was looking forward to experiencing sound performances live again while meeting many of my friends in person after times of social isolation during the COVID-19 pandemic. With consideration of the legal Corona measures at the time—a query of vaccination status, evidence of negative rapid testing, and the relocation to an outdoor venue—the festival enabled a sense of collectivity that had undergone immense changes and restrictions during the height of the pandemic. These were restrictions on social contact that, on the one hand, made people aware of an increased need for collectivity through deprivation, and, on the other hand, prevented physical collectivity and the spread of contagion for life-saving reasons.

---

1   It was especially because of the loving and devoted work and curation by Sandy Brede that the festival *Acting in Concert* became such a memorable event. Thank you for making a special time possible. Also thanks to Tubi, Mev, Manischa, Leah and the soft spot collective for the caring time there. I would also like to take this opportunity to thank Henriette Gunkel for her terrific comments and help in preparing this article. Without our sessions of thinking together, this article would not have come into being.

The danger of virus transmission through the exchange of aerosols extends the boundaries of (felt) corporeality. Airborne particles passing out of bodies into other bodies move by respiratory processes; in other words breathing. During the COVID-19 pandemic it was necessary to prevent close, shared breathing in order to avoid shortness of breath, which could be caused by infection. Thus, the bodily practice of breathing became visible especially when its (sometimes life-threatening) disruption was at stake. This becoming visible not only emphasizes the transgressiveness of bodies, the moving in and out of suspended particles across bodily boundaries, but also reveals that essential breathing is not made possible for all people in the same way. The examination of breathing therefore opens up questions about the availability of breathable air and about structural policies that allow certain bodies to breathe differently (Górska 2016). In his article "The Universal Right to Breathe" (2020), Achille Mbembe interweaves thoughts on breathing with the COVID-19 pandemic and calls for a "giant rupture" to end both the virological crisis and the long-standing structures of racism. During the coronavirus crisis, disciplinary measures and the call for "self-discipline, in a Foucauldian fashion, through social distancing" (Lee 2020) have become life-essential—and yet certain lives have been deliberately left to die.

The COVID-19 pandemic revealed a necropolitics of the kind described by Mbembe in 2003, one that reached a particular intensity in the wake of the pandemic (Lee 2020; Sandset 2021; Mbembe 2003 and 2020). The concept of necropolitics is characterized by a particular understanding of sovereignty whose ultimate expression, Mbembe argues, lies in the power to decide who may live and who must die. Or, in his own words: Necropolitics are "contemporary forms of subjugation of life to the power of death" (2003, 39). Mbembe's opposition to a classical understanding of sovereignty, which often associates sovereignty with nation states and state institutions, works with Foucault's concept of biopower, but questions whether it is sufficient to understand certain political and state violence, especially in light of technologies of racism (12):

> That race (or for that matter racism) figures so prominently in the calculus
> of biopower is entirely justifiable. After all, more so than class-thinking (the
> ideology that defines history as an economic struggle of classes), race has
> been the ever-present shadow in Western political thought and practice,
> especially when it comes to imagining the inhumanity of, or rule over, for-
> eign peoples. ... Indeed, in Foucault's terms, racism is above all a technology

aimed at permitting the exercise of biopower, 'that old sovereign right of death.' In the economy of biopower, the function of racism is to regulate the distribution of death and to make possible the murderous functions of the state. It is, he says, 'the condition for the acceptability of putting to death.' (17)

Mbembe derives necropower historically from the violent systems of the plantations, the former colonies, and apartheid to understand the subjugation of life to the power of death. He thus describes necropolitical structures that existed before the pandemic but these also became visible during COVID-19. Tony Sandset, for example, explains how the concept of necropolitics can show us "how health disparities and the COVID-19 pandemic has produced conditions not for living but for dying" (2021, 1411). By referring to Christopher J. Lee's reasoning that COVID-19 is foremost a crisis of sovereignty (2020), Sandset argues that "[t]he COVID-19 pandemic is entangled with necropolitical factors of slow violence and death that preceded the pandemic and adds to the disproportionate distribution of vulnerabilities towards the risk of infection, death, and economic impoverishment" (2021, 1412).

In the midst of this oppressive climate of cutting off breath and the simultaneous media confrontation with global injustices primarily affecting Black, Asian and Minority Ethnic (BAME) Communities, queer and disabled persons, there was the opportunity to visit a festival that announced itself to be "a place of retreat for many people—against a violent normative, racist, patriarchal and capitalist world" (Acting in Concert 2021a). Thus, attending *Acting in Concert* was also a search for bodily proximity, for a sense of collectivity in times of the pandemic. *Acting in Concert* became a utopian moment of safe collective perception, which retrospectively marks the starting point of this article.

In this article, I will investigate the politics of breath in light of the COVID-19 pandemic and as set out by Mbembe's return to necropolitics in this context and explore the question of "whose lives are breathable and whose loss of breath is grievable" (Górska 2016, 30) in relation to the festival and its performances. I am particularly interested in the affective forms of resistance to the necropolitics of breathing by focusing on sound performance and the scream, understood as a movement from the body, the sounding breath of a breathing body. The possibility to breathe and not to be suffocated as a "target body" is in fact the basic condition to have a voice and thus also to release a "sonorous-affective force" (Thompson 2013, 147). This force also became perceptible in the significant, resistant screams of the Black Lives Matter movement, in which voices were raised in response to the direct choking of George Floyd's breath. During the festival, the performance of the artist Iceboy Violet revealed a screaming voice protesting anti-Black and anti-queer violence. In the examination of Iceboy Violet's performance, screams are to be interrogated as auditory movements of disturbance. I will argue that there are certain sounds that reveal and mark themselves in particular ways as part of an environment and as part of bodies that have a particular affective impact as moments of disruptive exposure. In doing so, I also want to make clear that bodies are differently situated in environments. Contrary to a displacement of sonic events into an abstracted environment as independent sound without situated ground, the affecting scream will be thought of in political and environmental terms. Drawing on Black studies and Fred Moten's remarks on the particular qualities of sound in a Black Radical tradition, I will consider that the preconditions of Black bodies to affect with their art is altered by a historical lineage of structural violence and thus requires and produces different perceptual dispositifs than those that are supposedly universal. Based on Frantz Fanon's thesis that the Black male body does not form an ontological resistance, Moten develops the approach of an ontology of relation or movement. Blackness would thus take place in social death or non-being due to racism, but at the same time forms a movement/unrest that escapes this dehumanization. What occurs is a kind of spatial, paraontological unrest. I will read the contemporary sound performance of Iceboy Violet in the light of Moten's paraontological unrest. In addition to my experience of Iceboy Violet's live performance, I will also reference video works to enable different encounters with the sound of the scream. At this point I would like to emphasize that my engagement with the topic of systemic, violent, racializing structures and the attempt to perceive existing powerful disturbances is addressed from my white, Eurocentric perspective. This also means repeatedly reminding myself that the possible disruptive potentials of sound as paraontological unrest, its meaning, creation, and becoming interrogated here transcends my perspective and that underlying the sound works and theoretical ideas are experiences of violence that are not mine. Especially in Black studies, from the well-known work of Frederick Douglass to recent publications by Sadiya Hartmann and Fred Moten, the question arises how racist violence towards Black people can be addressed without creating a spectacle moment or further stigmatizing Black people as objectified victims. Can the scream as an affective force represent a possibility to escape this violent repetition while forming resistance and as such a sense of empowerment or agency of marginalized artists, especially People of Color?

## Deep Breathing, "U Don't Know My Name, U Don't Know My Name"

With a microphone in their hand, the Manchester-based sound artist, producer and vocalist Iceboy Violet began to speak, greeting the audience in a soft voice as they stepped down from the stage and stood among the crowd in a circle that was forming. Even before their performance, Iceboy Violet looked attentively at all the visitors and, with their consent, hugged the people who approached them. Then, Iceboy Violet went to the mixer, started the music and spoke. Their words became spoken word and formed a hybrid with the drone scapes that began to accelerate ever more noisily. There were serious but also warm words, that revealed Iceboy Violet's sensitivity and addressed their experience of hate crimes, violence, discrimination and exclusion as a trans* person of color. Looking up repeatedly, they gasped, took deep breaths, and rapped in grime style, shouting cautionary words to the environment. "It's cold outside, it's cold outside. But it's warm when I'm with you" (IMPA TV 2020). Positioned in the middle of the crowd, Iceboy Violet turned onlookers into empathizers, transforming the audience into a community at eye level, while at the same time the noise sound powerfully accompanied their screaming voice. Cries of grief and shouts of rage alternated with sounds of exhaustion and were accompanied by electronic sounds that seemed to offer a rhythm giving support. The sound performance effected what the festival site had announced before: "Iceboy Violet channels the energy, emotionality and resistance of grime. In doing so, fears, anger and defiance are given voice, functioning as a personal and collective catharsis" (Acting in Concert 2021b). This catharsis not only constituted Iceboy Violet as an emotional body, but also involved the audience's bodies and emotions in the performance in a unique way. The outcome were moments of sonic assemblage and an affect space that included the sobs and audible gasps for air from me and the affecting sounds of the other participants. There was a sense of special creativity, of affects that are not intrinsically constant, but that are connected and at work in this moment and this place. The understanding of affect here, then, refers primarily to the coming together of quasi-events and qualities as an assemblage in the moment of happening, without being universally valid. Such an *assemblage thinking* foregrounds a relational thinking in which "the endurant is not a thing that endures but the creativity of keeping in place something that is constantly changing. ... Nothing can ever be kept in place but can only be attended to" (Povinelli 2017, 182). Throughout Iceboy Violet's performance, an atmosphere was created that made a relational feeling between sadness, pain, anger and being touched briefly endurant, creating a space of collective affectivity. It was thus not a universal affect per se, but the creation of a terrain, a moving unrest that gave the emotion a brief effective permanence. Iceboy Violet created an environment for feeling, learning and for study as Fred Moten and Stefano Harney named it in *The Undercommons*: "Study is what you do with other people. It's talking and walking around with other people, working, dancing, suffering" (2013, 110).

During the performance, I perceived the people around me as similarly moved as I was; with tears in their eyes, hugging each other, supporting each other and/or Iceboy Violet. As Iceboy Violet describes it: "We talk about some horrible stuff, and then at the end, I walk through the audience and hug people, if they're comfortable with it. We're all coming to experience this together, so I try to end on something hopeful" (Iceboy Violet qtd. in McNulty 2022). The intensity of the performance and especially the affective space created by Iceboy Violet were stressful, hard to bear and uncomfortable and yet they contained moments of hope and empowerment—or, as the performer puts it themselves: "I try to make it so that you'll like it, but I'm not necessarily gonna make it comfortable" (qtd. in McNulty 2022). Iceboy Violet created a space of shared hurt, beyond spectacle and fetishization, in which emotions did not seem to be solely a personal belonging but became part of a shared affective event. Iceboy Violet confidently allowed the audience to share their personal and explicit experiences of pain, marked by racism and anti-queerness. But the performance also conveyed a pain that exists beyond Iceboy Violet's experience. A pain that is structural, that restricts, hurts and kills, became also part of the performance. But how did Iceboy Violet's performance, their screams manage to create an atmosphere that named a tradition of anti-Black and anti-queer violence, without reducing Iceboy Violet to a victim position to be mourned and thus further stigmatized?

In the first seconds of Iceboy Violet's performance in the video of *The Shape of Sound*, Iceboy Violet's deep amplified breathing is clearly audible (Somerset House 2019, 00:00:06–00:00:09). It is a breathing that auditorily invites intimacy, but also offers the intimacy of a lived experience; it is an offer to experience intimacy through sound. As Cathy Lane has argued in relation to the breathing in the performances of the multimedia artists Khaled Kaddal and Ansuman Biswas: "These works, which each focus on the breath in different ways, have invited the audience to share as powerfully an experience of emotional and physical intimacy as might be expected from sound." (Lane 2020, 208). The *Akademie der Künste*, referring to the works *Breath* and *Breathing Room* by the composer and artist Ain Bailey and the sound artist Hildegard Westerkamp similarly emphasize the community building capacity of sound performances: "This sound performance transforms the entirety of the space into a breathing organism . . . an immersive experience of visceral wake work" (Bailey 2018). In Iceboy Violet's live performance, there is a striking, sensitive breathing, a moaning integrated in echo effects and electronic tinkling sounds, also heard in the beginning of the video of the "Full Live Sets at *FAT OUT FEST 2020*" (IMPA TV 2020, 00:00:03–00:00:42).

Breathing is usually thought of as a self-evident, universal good and only receives attention at the moment of its disruption. Like a medium, breathing becomes perceptible when its process or mediation is disturbed, interrupted or curtailed; one literally loses one's breath. Beyond the unusually loud audible breathing, Iceboy Violet shouts and admonishes in their performance; they lament, grunt, and scream. These sounds can be heard particularly clearly in the video excerpts *Pieces* (IMPA TV 2020, 00:05:59–00:07:58), *Sceptic* (00:23:52–00:27:49) and *Vanity/Winner* (00:27:50–00:31:21). There are cries that sound differently, that are more than a mere transgression as discussed in Sound studies in relation to Noise Music. These cries and screams oscillate between grief, rage, and power and thus make it possible to experience moments of disturbance in a differentiated way. Sounds of breathing that are otherwise excluded from a performance because perceived as a disturbance[2] are performed and exposed here. When considering the process of making audible the supposedly imperceptible—silence or the noise of a background—under a lens of exposure, of exposition, instead of considering it solely as inappropriately noisy, as an undesirable, negative transgression, the noise carries a potential of empowered performance beyond standardized patterns of perception. This exposition operates beyond the norms of opposing taboos, that is, it transgresses or even dissolves boundaries. It does so by not following an

---

2    The subsequent removal of noise and other so-called unwanted sounds, such as audible breathing sounds, from the recorded signal is a common practice in the postproduction of recordings, whether in vocal pop song or podcast production. See, for example, the *Noise Gate* editing function. In addition, 'proper' breathing is a big part of professional vocal training.

effect of shock or fright alone, but by also revealing its own materiality and the process of its production. As Marie Suzanne Thompson puts it:

> Whilst noise music as transgression turns its ear to a transcendent and chaotic outside, as exposure it seeks a transformation of music from within. In this context, however, exposure is not simply an act of revelation but rather is a fundamentally creative act—an exploration of sonorous and affective potentials (we know not yet what noise can do). (2014, 207)

So, it is a sound that exposes itself by exhibiting its own supposed moment of disturbance, letting itself be felt. As the audience, we perceive what is not meant to be perceived in classical singing, for example, what is meant to be contained by breathing and recording techniques. The listeners become part of a border crossing in which the basic noise immanent in the system of recording and replay—here as vocal noise of a breathing process—demands perception as exposure. It is a scream for attention, an invitation to be affected. It is a voice that exhibits that it is part of a respiratory process and instead of letting it linger in imperceptibility as taken for granted, exposes it as a disturbance. In other words, the scream is "both about affect ... and is itself affective, insomuch that it seeks to mobilize other bodies by impacting upon their affective registers. The scream, as a sonorous-affective force, is thus responsible for the transference, or contagion of affects from one body to another" (Thompson 2013, 147). Understanding the scream as an affective force within an affective event makes it possible to think beyond its symbolic character and its representation as "a reflection of the unravelled psyche, the tortured, modern subject" (147). It is less about the question of what a scream *is*, but what it *does* or even *moves*. A sound as assertive as the scream opens up different levels of affect: on the one hand in the connotation with a state of suffering, with distress, panic, fear, pain or anger, and on the other hand as a cry of joy, as a positively excited outburst, as surprise or erotic-orgasmic expression. Whether screams of individuals or collectives all of them initially describe auditory moments with an immensely high affective capacity.

## Losing One's Breath and Voice

The cry, a moan or murmur, the shriek or wail, all these words comprise descriptions of different forms of auditory expression. In a first association, they stand out as possible forms of emotional communication, as a medium that makes pain, grief, shock, or joy perceptible. They appear as a medium that gives expression to an altered bodily sensation. On the one hand they are perceptible as auditory expressions of the body, on the other hand they are themselves audible embodiments. As an ensemble of vocal sounds, screams are a communicating medium that can be sent or received from one body to another, but also a quality that suggests that the body itself is a medium. Screams are a performative act of the voice.

But what does having a voice to scream require and what is the relationship to breathing? How do voices become audible and whose voices are heard? The voice as an interface between the body and its environment marks an audible movement in which something internal is carried into an external. It is a movement that takes place between two elastic vocal cords and an opening between them that mobilizes air, which, coming from the lungs, sets vibrations in motion, in turn materializing a sound that emerges into the outside. It is a sound that becomes tone, noise or sonority through air. It is a movement that aurally reveals that a voice is based on a breathing body and thus also marks the body as a respiratory system. But what happens when this movement stops, because the body literally runs out of breath? The basic prerequisite for a voice is respiration, a metabolic process that circulates air in a process of gaseous exchange across bodily boundaries with its surroundings, the environment. This process connects the body to its environment and air which itself, as a gas mixture of the earth's atmosphere, consists mainly of nitrogen and oxygen (Horn 2018). Air surrounds us, is elemental, connects the global and the local and "is a hybrid between human politics, scientific knowledge, and processes of nature" (8). Eva Horn thus speaks of "air as medium," and John Durham Peters of air as an "elemental media" (Peters 2015). With Peters and Horn's broader understanding of media in mind, which involves means by which worlds and habitats are created, I think of air, breathing and atmosphere as environmental and therefore understand media as environmental media (cf. Peters 2018, 179). Or as Horn puts it:

> An apprehension of *being in the air* thus means a heightened sense not just of our 'environments,' be they natural, social, urban, cultural, and so on; it actually means going beyond the divide between organism and environment towards a consciousness of our exchanges with it—the ways we breathe it, feel it on our skin, sweat and shiver, notice the smells and changes of the seasons. (Horn 2018, 19)

A sharpening of the senses with regard to the environment and a greater awareness of the fact that the body exists in exchange with its environment also needs to take into account, however, that not all organisms and subjects are influenced by the environment in the same way. It is thus precisely the examination of breathing that became central in the COVID-19 pandemic which opens up questions about the availability of breathable air, articulated by Mbembe (2020). Relating back to the writings of Frantz Fanon, Mbembe's work is situated in a postcolonial tradition of thinking about breathing. As early as 1952, Fanon, who gained attention as an important figure of postcolonial theory through his influential writings *Black Skin, White Mask* (1952) and *The Wretched of the Earth* (1961), opens up a space to reflect on the meaning and capacities of breathing in the course of colonialism:

> For Fanon, breath was at once a marker of epistemological occupation—'an observed, an occupied breathing' that formed part of the 'dependency complex' that justified colonisation—and the cause of revolt against it. It is not because the Indo-Chinese has discovered a culture of his own that he is in revolt. It is because 'quite simply' it was, in more than one way, becoming impossible for him to breathe. (Adams 2021)

Fanon's works address the brutality of state violence against marginalized, rebellious bodies, the systematic suffocation of those who dared to rise up and thus caused an increasingly global movement of revolt ([1952] 1967; cf. Adams 2021). In a global system marked by imperialist exploitation, Eurocentrism and racism, breathing as an environmental process becomes the site where structural power relations influence bodies and lives. Fanon thus counters the common assumption that every living being has the same capacities of breathing and that the possibilities to breathe are equally distributed. Instead, he describes an existing imbalance, a risk of not being able to breathe to which certain subjects (especially Black and Brown people) are exposed, which also includes the danger of suffocation as a systemic threat. Breathing is fleeting, elusive, barely visible, ephemeral, but has an elemental dimension and thus must be understood as an *event*. Fanon hence understands colonialism as a moment of respiration, an event in which the outside is let into the inside, along with all its violence. He conceives colonialism as a form of social metabolic process in which the political is seen as a transformation of the body in relation to the environment. This also means that the political marks a relationship between one's body and its environment. While the respective organic processes of breathing are universal, they are nevertheless deeply connected to the specific context in which breathing is performed. In his critique of the French colonization of Algeria in his 1965 work *Combat Breathing*, Fanon describes how breathing and spatiality, breathing and politics, embodiment and subjectivity, individual situatedness and power structures are interrelated (cf. Górska 2016, 276). He writes: "There is not occupation of territory, on the one hand, and independence of persons on the other. It is the country as a whole, its history, its daily pulsation that are contested, disfigured, in the hope of a final destruction. Under these conditions, the individual's breathing is an observed, an occupied breathing. It is a combat breathing" (Fanon 1965, 65). *Combat Breathing* illustrates the extent to which social power relations are characterized by 'suffocating operations' and require those affected to breathe for survival. According to Suvendrini Perera and Joseph Pugliese in reference to Fanon, a "target body" is "reduced to a soma of such utter political and economic vulnerability that the very possibility of respiration becomes the ultimate challenge. As such, the target subject's energies are fully committed merely to surviving" (2011, 2). The logic of state violence engages the 'target subject' in 'breathing for survival,' leaving them with no energies to question their situation or to resist. In resistance, the connection between breathing and voice also becomes perceptible: breathing is the basic prerequisite for a voice; that is, it is only through breathing that it becomes possible to have a voice. Through colonialism, which hinders or prevents access to breathing, access to the voice is also distributed unequally. The voice, in turn, is essential for various forms of protest, thus: making it impossible to breathe also makes voice-based resistance impossible.

There are various restrictions to breathing, access to good, clean air to breathe being one of them. Air pollution is one of the most dangerous effects of the climate catastrophe and does not affect all people equally. It often affects people who do not cause it, both on an international and on a national level. For example, in the context of the USA, studies highlight so-called *environmental racism*, which means that in certain regions, Black People, Indigenous People and People of Color (BIPoC) in particular are affected by environmental pollution as well as air pollution because they are pushed into environments that are hostile to life (Alves 2014; Carter, Butler, and Dwyer 2011; McKittrick 2006; Neimanis, Åsberg, and Hedrén 2015; Ramirez 2015; Wilson 2000; Wright 2021). There are also more direct restrictions of breathing: In 2020, for example, in the USA, George Floyd was pinned down on the ground by a police officer to the point where he screamed "I can't breathe" and eventually died from this restriction to his breathing. His murder led to huge protests by the Black Lives

Matter movement in the USA and beyond which formed on the streets at the height of the COVID-19 pandemic despite the need/demand/politics for social distancing. It remains indeed remarkable how millions of people protested together in the streets, even before a vaccine was developed, thus despite the increased risk of contracting the deadly virus which, in the USA, Black and Brown people were disproportionally effected by. As Ed Pilkington observes in *The Guardian:* "Across the country, African Americans have died at a rate of 50.3 per 100,000 people, compared with 20.7 for whites, 22.9 for Latinos and 22.7 for Asian Americans" (2020). COVID-19 is a disease that also makes it impossible for many of those infected to breathe on their own and which particularly affected and still affects (multiple) marginalized people who often have less access to health care because of their social status/ social position.[3] The idea of combat breathing, as set out by Fanon in the specific context of colonialism, thus extends into the present where police brutality as well as the COVID-19 pandemic make visible that breathing remains an environmental and highly political process and as such the precondition of (collective) resistance. In the final section of this chapter, I will explore this further by turning to Moten's concept of troubled air and the resistant, non-figurative potential of the scream as 'sonorous-affective forces' in the context of anti-blackness.

## Troubled Air and the Scream as Resistance

"Moten's troubled air is what escapes when blackness (as object, as commodity, as non-being) is both enforced and refused, arising through the vibration of the object against its frame. The troubled air of the black object that resists its existence as such might be a screech or a scream." (Thompson 2017, 278)

Audible protests, cut off breath, a virus-laden environment portray a climate of turbulence—an environment of troubled air. It is a hostile climate that also contains movements that rebel against the oppression, that scream in resistance. But does the experience of Iceboy Violet's screams resemble the paraontological power of the screams that are significant in Moten's and

---

3     Germain and Yong (2020) describe barriers to health care arising e.g. from racist medical beliefs, cultural barriers related to gender, including information barriers and stigma, and legal barriers arising from immigration law and status.

Thompson's remarks? Considering screams of resistance as 'sonorous-affective forces' within performances of a sound event that moves and is not to
be confused with an understanding of sound that asserts an undifferenti-
ated immediacy of sound, I will subsequently illustrate that the ontological
has to be located in the political. Ontologies are characterized by "racialised
erasures and exclusions from the realm of ontology" (Thompson 2017, 268).
Sylvia Wynter has demonstrated how "ontological accounts of the human
emerge with colonial conquest; and how being, subsequently, is equated with
the overrepresented ethnoclass of Western, bourgeois man, resulting in the
obfuscation of other modes and possibilities of being" (2003, 267). The colonial
history of race/racialization and slavery, according to Fanon, prevents a Black
being from being included in a white-defined realm of being; that is, Blackness would be relegated to a field of non-being, which would also 'suffocate' an
equivalent capacity for action. Fred Moten contradicts and expands Fanon's
idea that Black being is characterized by an ontological non-being; instead, he
sees the possibility for paraontological resistance. Within the framework of
a paraontology of disorder, Moten speaks of 'objects of resistance' of a Black
radical tradition. Blackness is paraontological in that the lived experience of
Blackness can both enact and escape the assignment of Blackness to social
death, to a state of non-being. Being, or the lived experience (of Blackness), is
thus not—as Fanon points out—something static, but something in motion.
In this sense, Iceboy Violet's moving cries, their growls and moans are thought
of as "troubled air" (Moten 2008, 182). In the song DEATHDRIVE (IMPA TV
2020, 00:23:52–00:27:49) Iceboy Violet begins with echoing words embedded
in melodic carpets of noise. Words like 'why' and 'from the hole' multiply as rep-
etitions of the echo and spread out in the space like waves (00:23:53–00:24:10).
Iceboy Violet thematizes a being in the depths that does not linger, remains
static "in the hole," but takes up pace. It is a drive close to death, a non-being
in the social life but at the same time they remind their audience, "I am still
here" (00:24:19). There are screeching voices in the background as Iceboy Violet
contorts their face, but then catches their breath, stretches and groans, "yeah"
(00:24:53). After a moment of gathering strength Iceboy Violet's angry and
empowering screams follow from 00:24:59 onwards. The smashing sonorous-
affective forces "crush our system daily" (00:25:19) and culminate in their cries
for reassurance and self-assertion: "I'm still alive, I'm still alive, I will survive"
(00:25:50–00:26:00). The performance is characterized by forces spreading
between non-being and being, it is a troubled air of disturbance, which Moten
describes as "an irruption of phonic substance" (2003, 14). It is a movement that

appears spatially, which makes resistance possible. It is a paraontolology and thus a moment of recurrent Black being, a "becoming-object of the speaking, singing, commodified object" (Moten 2017, 33). Iceboy Violet's breathy voice moves through space, producing chaos that creates its own speaking space.

In this space, a pain becomes present which points towards the historical lineage of structural violence against People of Color. Iceboy Violet created a space that holds their own screams, but also, as I would argue, the screams of Frederick Douglass's Aunt Hester whose screams have become a starting point for debates on the reproduction of anti-Black violence in Black studies. In his autobiographical book *Narrative of the Life of Frederick Douglass* (1845)[4], Douglass, born into slavery in the United States in Maryland, describes a scene in which his aunt Hester is beaten and whipped. The screams of his aunt Hester were the first glimpse into the cruelty of slavery for him and hence symbolic of the violence of the system of slavery and the total, brutal subjugation of the enslaved. The screams explicitly described by Douglass, caused by the blows of a tormentor, are the ones that Moten marks as a 'primal scene'/'inaugural moment' in his response to an analysis by the literary and cultural scholar Saidiya Hartman. Hartman draws on Douglass' retellings of this violence to critique how the reproduction of such scenes of violence against the enslaved body can turn into spectacles of Black suffering (cf. Hartman 1997, 4).[5] Moten, in response, questions whether an avoidance of the representation of violence by not naming it is possible at all—if violence exists as a primal scene and he suggests that performance might function beyond economies of reproduction. He is interested in showing that performances—especially those situated in a Black radical tradition—have their own energies, opportunities and potentials inherent in their re-performance as presence and disturbance. In this sense, Iceboy Violet's performance can be understood as reproducing violence by making pain tangible,

---

4    The book is considered to be one of the most influential works of the American abolitionist movement.

5    Through the reproduction of violent scenes, there is often an approximate familiarity with them, reinforcing a spectacle-becoming of Black suffering. Hartman responds to such unintended familiarity in her own writing, in *Scenes of Subjection*, by explaining and stating that she does not want to reproduce the violence that happened to Aunt Hester. Instead of a suffering Black body, Hartman wants to emphasize an 'everydayness' in order to avoid a repeated reproduction of violence and the re-enactment of the objectification of Black bodies: "Does this not reinforce the 'thingly' quality of the captive by reducing the body to evidence in the very effort to establish the humanity of the enslaved?" (1997, 19).

by not avoiding it, but by embedding it in an interaction between presence and disturbance. It is precisely the interplay between reproduction and disappearance that constitutes the condition and ontology of performance in the first place (Moten 2003, 5).

In a turbulent environment of a pandemic that intensified the conditions of the necropolitical deathdrive, the systematic restriction of the breath of the marginalized, the reproduction of the extreme violence against George Floyd—his suffocation—became an important point of reference for the Black Lives Matter movement. The engagement with Iceboy Violet's performance, with their over-present breathing, screaming and moaning, aimed to show that possible objects of resistance in contemporary performances can enable a thematization of unspeakable anti-Black violence that oscillates between presence and disturbance. In Iceboy Violet's (live) performance, a violence was made perceptible and tangible that did not seem to surrender to any totalizing effect or left a victim without agency. On the contrary: Iceboy Violet speaks out, has a voice that, in spite of the structural restriction to their breathing—especially during the COVID-19 Pandemic—produces resistance. In the shared experience at the festival, affect assemblages emerged as screams, inviting collective perseverance in emotions that seemed to materialize an opening to confront the rage and grief of an agonizing history in community. Oscillating between endurance and violation, Iceboy Violet performs in a Black tradition as described by Moten. Thus, they thematizes and performs a pain that was already part of Frederick Douglass Aunt Hester's screams. It is not the whipping that is the moment of reproduction, but the scream as paraontological unrest. The scream as an expression became an intersection of the politics of breathing, voice and auditory movement. Read as paraontological unrest, screams enable movements that open a space to call attention to a structural violence by making visible and audible a lived experience of Blackness between reproduction and subversion. Within necropolitical, breath-taking structures—which have become particularly visible during the pandemic—the scream can be a disturbance that is resistant.

## Works Cited

Acting in Concert. 2021a. "Acting in Concert Festival 2021." *Acting in Concert*, Accessed May 30, 2023. https://actinginconcert.org/acting-in-concert-festival-2021.

Acting in Concert. 2021b. "Iceboy Violet." *Acting in Concert*, Accessed May 30, 2023. https://actinginconcert.org/Iceboy-Violet.

Adams, Ross Exo. 2021. "On Breath: Breathing in the Cloud." *Platform Austria*, 2021. Last Accessed May 30, 2023. https://www.platform-austria.org/en/b log/on-breath-breathing-in-the-cloud.

Alves, Jaime Amparo. 2014. "From Necropolis to Blackpolis: Necropolitical Governance and Black Spatial Praxis in São Paulo, Brazil." *Antipode* 46, no. 2 (March): 323–39. https://doi.org/10.1111/anti.12055.

Bailey, Ain. 2018. "Breath: Koloniales Erbe." *Akademie der Künste*, May 26, 2018. https://www.adk.de/de/projekte/2018/koloniales-erbe/symposium-II/programm/breath.htm.

Carter, Perry L., David Butler, and Owen Dwyer. 2011. "Defetishizing the Plantation: African Americans in the Memorialized South." *Historical Geography* 39, no. 2 (January): 128–46.

Douglass, Frederick. 1845. *Narrative of the Life of Frederick Douglass: An American Slave, Written by Himself*. Boston: Anti-Slavery Office.

Fanon, Frantz. (1952) 1967. *Black Skin, White Masks*. Translated by Charles Lam Markmann. New York: Grove Press.

———. (1961) 1968. *The Wretched of the Earth*. Translated by Constance Farrington. New York: Grove Press.

Germain, Sabrina, and Adrienne Yong. 2020. "COVID-19 Highlighting Inequalities in Access to Healthcare in England: A Case Study of Ethnic Minority and Migrant Women." *Feminist Legal Studies* 28: 301–10.

Górska, Magdalena. 2016. *Breathing Matters: Feminist Intersectional Politics of Vulnerability*. Linköping: Linköping University Electronic Press.

Hartman, Saidiya. 1997. *Scenes of Subjection: Terror, Slavery, and Self-Making in Nineteenth-Century America*. Oxford: Oxford University Press.

Horn, Eva. 2018. "Air as Medium." *Grey Room* 73 (Fall): 6–25.

IMPA TV. 2020. "IMPATV 256—Iceboy Violet—Full Set Live at Fat Out Fest 2020." Uploaded November 20, 2020. YouTube, https://www.youtube.com /watch?v=DUGl1HrLXNs.

Interkultureller Kalender. "Die Unsicherheit aushalten. Ein Gespräch mit Sandy Brede (acting in concert) | Interkultur Ruhr." 2022. https://interkul tur.ruhr/notiz/die-unsicherheit-aushalten-ein-gespraech-mit-sandy-bre de-acting-in-concert.

Lane, Cathy. 2020. "Gender, Intimacy, and Voices in Sound Art: Encouragments, Self-Portraits, and Shadow Walks." In *The Bloomsbury Handbook of*

*Sound Art,* edited by Sanne Groth and Holger Schulze, 198–212. New York: Bloomsbury Academic.

Lee, Christopher J. 2020. "The Necropolitics of COVID-19." *Africa Is a Country,* April 1, 2020. https://africasacountry.com/2020/04/the-necropolitics-of-c ovid-19.

Mbembe, Achille. 2003. "Necropolitics." Translated by Libby Meintjes. *Public Culture* 15, no. 1 (January): 11–40. https://doi.org/10.1215/08992363-15-1-11.

———. 2020. "The Universal Right to Breathe." Translated by Carolyn Shread. *Critical Inquiry* 47, no. S2: 58–62. https://doi.org/10.1086/711437.

McKittrick, Katherine. 2006. *Demonic Grounds: Black Women and the Cartographies of Struggle.* Minnesota: University of Minnesota Press.

McNulty, Sophie. 2022. "Get to Know: Iceboy Violet." *DJ Mag.* May 30, 2022. ht tps://djmag.com/features/get-know-iceboy-violet.

Moten, Fred. 2003. *In the Break: The Aesthetics Of The Black Radical Tradition.* Minnesota: University of Minnesota Press.

———. 2008. "The Case of Blackness." *Criticism* 50, no. 2 (Spring): 177–218. htt ps://doi.org/10.1353/crt.0.0062.

———. 2017. *Black and Blur.* Durham: Duke University Press.

Neimanis, Astrida, Cecilia Åsberg, and Johan Hedrén. 2015. "Four Problems, Four Directions for Environmental Humanities: Toward Critical Posthumanities for the Anthropocene." *Ethics and the Environment* 20, no. 1 (Spring): 67–97. https://doi.org/10.2979/ethicsenviro.20.1.67.

Patterson, Orlando. 1982. *Slavery and Social Death.* Cambridge: Harvard University Press.

Perera, Suvendrini, and Joseph Pugliese. 2011. "Introduction: Combat Breathing. State Violence and the Body in Question." *Somatechnics* 1, no. 1: 1–14.

Peters, John Durham. 2015. *The Marvelous Clouds: Toward a Philosophy of Elemental Media.* Chicago: University of Chicago Press.

———. 2018. "The Media of Breathing." In *Atmospheres of Breathing,* edited by Lenart Skof and Petri Berndtson, 179–98. New York: SUNY Press.

Pilkington, Ed. 2020. "Black Americans Dying of Covid-19 at Three Times the Rate of White People." *The Guardian.* May 20, 2020. https://www.theguard ian.com/world/2020/may/20/black-americans-death-rate-covid-19-coro navirus.

Povinelli, Elizabeth A., Mathew L. Coleman, and Kathryn Yusoff. 2017. "An Interview with Elizabeth Povinelli: Geontopower, Biopolitics and the Anthropocene." *Theory, Culture & Society* 34, no. 2–3: 169–85. https://doi.org/10.1177/0263276417689900.

Ramirez, Margarete Marietta. 2015. "The Elusive Inclusive: Black Food Geographies and Racialized Food Spaces." *Antipode* 47, no. 3: 748–69.

Roberts, Neil. 2015. *Freedom as Marronage*. Chicago: University of Chicago Press.

Sandset, Tony. 2021. "The Necropolitics of COVID-19: Race, Class and Slow Death in an Ongoing Pandemic." *Global Public Health* 16, no. 8/9 (March): 1411–23. https://doi.org/10.1080/17441692.2021.1906927.

Somerset House. 2019. "Iceboy Violet: The Shape of Sound." Uploaded January 17, 2019. YouTube, https://www.youtube.com/watch?v=tnGVV8NEOw8.

Thompson, Marie. 2013. "Three Screams." In *Sound, Music, Affect: Theorizing Sonic Experience*, edited by Marie Thompson and Ian Biddle, 147–62. London: A&C Black.

———. 2017. "Whiteness and the Ontological Turn in Sound Studies." *Parallax* 23, no. 3: 266–82. https://doi.org/10.1080/13534645.2017.1339967.

Thompson, Marie Suzanne. 2014. "Beyond Unwanted Sound: Noise, Affect and Aesthetic Moralism." PhD. diss., Newcastle University. Bloomsbury Publishing EBooks.

Wilson, Bobby M. 2000. *America's Johannesburg: Industrialization and Racial Transformation in Birmingham*. Lanham, Maryland: Rowman & Littlefield Publishers.

Wright, Willie Jamaal. 2021. "As Above, So Below: Anti-Black Violence as Environmental Racism." *Antipode* 53, no. 3: 791–809. https://doi.org/10.1111/anti.12425.

Wynter, Sylvia. 2003. "Unsettling the Coloniality of Being/Power/Truth/Freedom: Towards the Human, After Man, Its Overrepresentation—An Argument." *CR: The New Centennial Review* 3, no. 3 (Fall): 257–337. https://doi.org/10.1353/ncr.2004.0015.

# 11. Re-Negotiating Discourses on AIDS during the COVID-19 Pandemic: A Roundtable Discussion

*Simon Dickel, Roselyne Masamha, Lennon Mhishi, and Florian Zitzelsberger*
*Questions and Introduction: Heike Steinhoff*

The call for papers for the symposium that turned into this volume solicited a strikingly high number of contributions that addressed the HIV/AIDS crisis of the 1980s and 1990s and its (in)comparability to the COVID-19 pandemic of the 2020s. This sparked the idea of a roundtable discussion on this topic that allows for a variety of different perspectives on the topic and sets these into relation with one another. In the following, four scholars from different backgrounds offer their thoughts and arguments in response to three questions that address the (non-)relations of HIV/AIDS and SARS-CoV-2 /COVID-19 in regards to processes of othering.

In conversation: Simon Dickel, Professor of Gender and Diversity, Roselyne Masamha, Clinical Educator and independent researcher and Lennon Mishi, anthropologist and project researcher at the Pitt Rivers Museum, Florian Zitzelsberger, research assistant of American Studies/Cultural and Media Studies.

Questions and conceptualization: Heike Steinhoff, Junior Professor of American Studies.

## In how far can pandemic narratives surrounding SARS-CoV-2/COVID-19 be linked to those surrounding HIV/AIDS?

**Florian Zitzelsberger:** AIDS has served as one of the backdrops for artistic reactions to COVID-19: For example, lockdown performances of AIDS drama—examples include Kushner's *Angels in America* (1991/1992) and Finn and Lapine's musical *Falsettos* (1992)—were released on YouTube in support of the Foundation for AIDS Research (amfAR) and the Actors Fund, respectively, collecting donations to further research on COVID-19 and in support of individuals in the performing arts. I have elsewhere proposed that digital collaborations like "Scenes from ANGELS IN AMERICA" and "Falsettos in Quarantine" highlight the possibilities of connecting with others at a moment when the assumed collective experience of time was not (or no longer) possible, which draws attention to the precariousness of the lives of those who have never been able to share this experience to begin with (Zitzelsberger 2022, 482–83). But why AIDS, and why now? For one, because pandemic times "reveal continuity with historical precedent" (Waterman 2020, 761), COVID-19 directs us back to AIDS as one of the most recent examples of a virus spreading with pandemic scope, even if the kind of transmission differs in the cases of HIV and SARS-CoV-2. In this sense, I identify a potential for the emergence of solidarity in witnessing AIDS drama during the COVID-19 pandemic, especially its early stages under the precept of social distancing, that goes beyond the idea of understanding or feeling the (temporal) other—which necessarily remains somewhat illusory—and puts us in touch with the isolation we ourselves may experience during the present pandemic (Zitzelsberger 2022, 482; 486).

Additionally, such a dialogue between AIDS and COVID-19 draws attention to the way specific groups are entangled with a virus, based on the moralization of the kind of transmission in the former case—with discussions mostly focusing on gay men and intravenous drug users—and the supposed origin of the airborne virus in China in the latter. In both cases, the discursive pathology of the people associated with a 'gay' or 'Chinese virus' becomes engrained in the fabric of society as an us-versus-them narrative that produces material, and medical, effects. While there is stigma attached to many diseases, the propensity to use disease to create dis-ease for those affected by it—by marking them as a common enemy—that we can witness during the COVID-19 pandemic echoes the repulsion with which U.S. society confronted the AIDS crisis in the 1980s and 1990s.

Since 2020, scholars and journalists alike have asked whether society has learned anything in almost 40 years between the pandemics regarding the impact of othering in the context of disease. I would suggest that such a question is misleading in that 'learning' is not an exclusive project of the past. As Shotwell (2014) contends, the question should rather extend to how the memory of AIDS "is used in crafting livable futures in the context of systemic and ongoing oppression" (513). And in this, we find a possible explanation as to why

AIDS, and why now: bringing back the memory of AIDS so prominently during COVID-19 not only serves as a reminder of the impact of othering on the (psychic) survival of those affected by it. The work of remembering AIDS has significant bearing on how we circumvent the stigmatization and pathologization of people who contracted SARS-CoV-2 as well as those thought to be responsible for the spread of COVID-19. In turn, the experience of living through the COVID-19 pandemic shapes this memory—or the ways in which we allow ourselves to remember past pandemics—and can become a source of solidarity. AIDS narratives can serve as a foil for our very own COVID-19 narratives: They become a site of cross-temporal exchange where the mechanisms and consequences of othering can be interrogated. Looking at the AIDS crisis with what we know now, we might similarly be able to reflect on the present and imagine possible futures in which solidarity prevails. The dialogue between AIDS and COVID-19 demonstrates that we cannot move beyond othering if we keep letting the metaphors that killed in the past, to adopt Sontag's (2002, 99) poignant phrasing, kill in the present.

**Simon Dickel:** The lockdown performances Florian Zitzelsberger names are but two examples out of a very large number of performances people uploaded to the internet during COVID-19. Most of them covered different genres and topics and were generally unrelated to HIV/AIDS. Even though the producers of the performance of *Angels in America* quoted by Florian claim in the opening titles that they see a continuity from the AIDS crisis to COVID-19, the correlation of the two historical moments does not become apparent in the performance itself. I contend that the lockdown-performances of dramatic texts from other contexts rather point to the fact that there has not been a significant number of original artistic reactions to COVID-19. No texts comparable to the numerous radical, immediate, and urgent texts negotiating the AIDS crisis come to mind. This absence of artistic responses to COVID-19 is a good thing, because it attests to the different historical situations of the two pandemics, which are incommensurable. Narratives surrounding COVID-19 should therefore not be linked to those surrounding AIDS.

The long governmental neglect of the AIDS-crisis revealed a fundamental social misrecognition and shaming of gay men, sex workers, and IV-drug users. The misrecognition also becomes apparent in the obstacles the surviving lovers and friends encountered when mourning those who died from AIDS. In the literature of the 1980 and 90s, we find many examples that show how the biological families of those who died from AIDS took charge of the funeral rites, excluded the dead person's circle of friends, and altered the official cause of death. What is more, official recognition, such as memorials or rituals of public mourning to remember those who died from AIDS, was completely absent in the first years of the pandemic. In light of this misrecognition, activists had to invent new forms of public memory, and the Names Project AIDS memorial quilt and the political funerals of 'ACT UP' are two well-known examples.

The failure to publicly recognize those who died from AIDS points to the fact that their lives were not grievable. In *Frames of War: When is Life Grievable*, Judith Butler explains how the value of a life and its grievability are related: "Precisely because a living being may die, it is necessary to care for that being so that it may live. Only under conditions under which the loss would matter does the value of the life appear" (2016, 14). She explicitly refers to the Names Project and points out how it "broke through the public shame associated with dying from AIDS, a shame associated sometimes with homosexuality, and especially anal sex, and sometimes with drugs and promiscuity. It meant something to state and show the name, to put together some remnants of a life, to publicly display and avow the loss" (39).

In the context of COVID-19 the situation was decidedly different. From the beginning of the pandemic and in stark contrast to the AIDS crisis, lives lost to COVID-19 have always been grievable lives, and an infection with COVID-19 was not related to stigmatization and shame. The state ceremonies and numerous public memorials demonstrate the social recognition of those infected with COVID-19. I would like to clarify that I do not want to diminish the severity of anti-Asian racism in the context of COVID-19. It demonstrates the alarming fact that racist views are widely held and how easily they can be activated. I do agree with Florian Zitzelsberger that such racism calls for solidarity and should be met by a political response.

**Roselyne Masamha and Lennon Mhishi:** This issue of grievable lives is an interesting one to explore, considering the shifting contexts shaping how one defines, understands, experiences, and inhabits a world (un)constituted by the 'grievable.' Not being able to see people as they transformed in how they were known, as relations, to being unwell, as patients, as confined, and as they died and not being able to hold/attend funerals of those who succumbed to COVID-19 may raise the question of the changing nature of the 'grievable.' In addition, we are also confronted with the narratives about infected so-called anti-vaxers or guidance breachers, whose dying words were stated to have been laments over their behavior. Leading to the associated conversations of those deserving and not deserving to be mourned, again challenging the issue of whose/which lives were considered grievable. Vaccine hesitancy also saw groups of people being seen as 'having brought it on themselves' if they caught the infection and died as a result—again the issue of 'grievability' is interesting to explore in this wider context of COVID-19.

The intertwinement of state-led narratives, a dominant common sense of responsibilization, and the aftermaths of lockdowns and transformations in how we encounter disease and death as mediated by the forms of information availed to us, means that we are still coming to terms with what it might mean to grieve. With the impacts of what has been termed 'long COVID' still being studied, there may yet be much more to grieve, and in different ways. The experiences of debilitation, loss, mourning and grief across pandemics demands that we attend to this grieving as intrinsic to these specific conjunctures, manifesting differently on the basis of the structures governing intimacy and other forms of human contact, and consequently feeling and the common sense of what grieving is, and who or what we must grieve for. In other words, the grief across time might be regarded as interminable (Cole 2015).

Recognizing the differences and specificities of the pandemics is as important as exploring echoes and nodes of connection from which better understanding can be drawn. In the manner that knowledge in a productive yet humble way can be incremental, with previous experience shaping new learning, past pandemics can be instructive in what or how not to do things, and whether we do, as the cliché goes, learn anything from our histories. The issue of stigma is a case in point, both HIV/AIDS and COVID-19 demonstrate how HIV/AIDS related stigma and COVID-19 related stigma operated along and intersect with existing patterns and practices of stigma.

Stigmatization and shame occurred with COVID-19 infections, depending on how the infection was perceived to have been contracted. When considering the 'super-spreader' narratives, the patient zero conversations about responsibility and blame. Furthermore, the use of shame as an instrument to order behavior, for example *'Save your grandma—you should be ashamed of the risk you are introducing through your selfish behaviour, Save the National Health Service'* strap lines in the UK were all used to shame people into adhering to guidance. Indeed, the phrase—*Shame on you*—was reiterated often.

HIV/AIDS and COVID-19 reflect the health, moral and racial dimensions of stigma (Goffman 1963) and are aligned with historical patterns of disease attribution (Jones 2020; Sontag 1978). Patterns of developing 'loose' theories or suggestive imagery that reinforces existing perspectives of disease other-ing, replicate themselves in similar ways across the two diseases. A now in-famous headline from a German newspaper reported following the Omicron variant, "Das Virus aus Afrika ist bei uns" (The virus from Africa is with us) and included a picture of a Black mother and a child to accompany the headline (Ihekweazu). This type of headline sits on a longstanding fault line which per-petuates the negative stereotype of Africans and disease, against Europeans and purity. More recently, The Foreign Press Association, Africa, issued a state-ment to push back against the use of images of black people to depict the out-break of monkey pox in Europe and America.

In a similar vein, these narratives apply to the gay population in terms of the aforementioned us-and-them divides which create diseased groups and victim groups. Monkeypox again more recently was situated as a disease amongst gay people, associations of disease with particular groups of people have been present historically with the naming, for example, in the early 1980s of the HIV/AIDS epidemic as Gay-Related Immune Deficiency (GRID). Such naming and associations give permanence to the issue of stigma, the World Health Organization deliberately named COVID-19 to avoid conflation with a location of origin, yet referrals to it as the "Chinese" and "Wuhan" virus persist (World Health Organization 2020).

To return to the initial question about how narratives of SARS-CoV-2/COVID-19 can be linked to those of HIV/AIDS, the use of these narratives to build on and extend an understanding of the complexity of stigma and its various dimensions would be a useful consideration.

## What are pitfalls of the comparison of SARS-CoV-2/COVID-19 and HIV/AIDS and where do you see narrative ruptures?

**Simon Dickel:** My statement on the pitfalls of comparing COVID and AIDS relates to North American and Western European contexts. I contend that the ways of sexual transmission of the HI-Virus and the cultural meanings attached to them complicate a parallel perspective on the two pandemics. The AIDS-crisis had a fundamental and long-lasting impact on sexual culture. Gay men were most severely affected, not only by the dire consequences of HIV/AIDS-diseases, and almost certain death before the advent of antiretroviral therapies, but also by the sex-negative and homophobic discourse, stigma-tization, and social misrecognition connected to HIV. The close connection of sex and death in the case of HIV/AIDS not only resonates with earlier sex-negative cultural narratives, it also is the reason why guilt and shame are linked to HIV. The German sexologist Martin Dannecker speaks of a phobia of the lived body ("Leibphobie") and an altered economy of desire and argues that HIV led to a fundamental change in how gay men understood themselves as sexual subjects (2022, 330). I would like to address the consequences of this experience of stigmatization in relation to Didier Eribon's notion of insult. His book *Insult and the Making of the Gay Self* ([1999] 2004) is motivated by the question, which effects insults have on the body and describes them as "traumatic events experienced more or less violently at the moment they happen, but that stay in memory and in the body (for fear, awkwardness, and shame are bodily attitudes produced by a hostile exterior world)" (15). Insults can determine the degree of freedom and agency with which gay men can inhabit the world. Eribon maintains that "one of the consequences of insult is to shape the relation one has to others and to the world and thereby to shape the personality, the subjectivity, the very being of the individual in question" (15). Building on Pierre Bourdieu's concept of habitus, which relates to class, he outlines a theory of sexual habitus.

Walt Odets's 2019 book *Out of the Shadows: Reimagining Gay Men's Lives* gives ample evidence of the relation between stigmatization and AIDS and of Dannecker's description of the fundamental change of the self-image of many gay men, which was caused by HIV/AIDS. The psychotherapist builds on decades of experience of therapeutic work with gay men. He maintains that to this day most gay men are severely affected by HIV. He states that across three generations "many gay men ... both positive and negative, experience shame about the very fact of the HIV epidemic—as if it confirmed the justice in broadly stigmatizing gay lives" (79). Stating that both pandemics are alike stands in the way of adequately remembering those who died of AIDS and makes it difficult to understand and honor the political achievements of activist groups, such as 'ACT UP.' Stating that COVID-19 is just like AIDS stands in the way of gay men of all generations who want to emancipate themselves from the ways in which stigmatization affects their bodily being in the world.

I am convinced that oral history projects, such as the 'ACT UP' Oral History Project conducted by Jim Hubbard and Sarah Schulman, the Swedish Face of AIDS Archive, or the European HIV/AIDS Archive are the resources needed to grasp the full dimensions of the first stage of the AIDS-crisis in the 1980s and 90s and its long-lasting effects. The testimonies in these archives support my point that HIV and SARS-CoV2 should be treated as incommensurable pandemics.

**Roselyne Masamha and Lennon Mhishi:**  At surface level, there are some similarities between the HIV/ AIDS and COVID-19 pandemics. However, comparisons between the two require careful understanding of the broader manifestations of the two pandemics, especially the specific experiences of different communities across the spectrum: gender, age, class, race.

Comparisons also similarly demand attention to the particular historical moment and circumstances within which these pandemics have been experienced. HIV and AIDS affected, in greater numbers and with more severity, groups of people who were already marginalized. We make particular reference here to homosexual individuals and racialized populations, the former group being constructed as a deviant sexual identity and the latter having identities steeped within the notion of carriers and purveyors of disease. Being perceived as embodiments of a 'deadly virus' further ostracized and reinforced both groups' 'pollutant' identities while eroding their connections with the wider public. This double negative identity, compounded by existent exclusions and lack of will both politically and scientifically, affected the efforts made to invest time and resources into understanding the disease, its effects and exploring treatment options.

Against this backdrop, combined with the chronic and prolonged spread over a more sustainable time frame with less pressure on healthcare systems; the acute nature of COVID-19 and its relatively short recovery time is in sharp contrast, making comparisons problematic. This with recognition of the growing acknowledgement of the chronic impact of 'long COVID' whose understanding is still in its infancy. For the most part, COVID-19's acute nature and generally widespread impact has meant that its effects have been realized in a relatively short period of time; therefore, leading to the greater and more readily acknowledged impact on individuals, communities and livelihoods. This then led to significant public health efforts, as well as funded research. On the other hand, for a significant part of the early and extended occurrence of HIV and AIDS, attention to the impact and need for intervention was mobilized more through activism and concerted efforts of community groups, in the absence of/with limited engagement of public health authorities and research funding. The result of this slow response continues to be felt across different populations with ongoing devastating effects.

The indiscriminate nature of the spread of COVID-19 has also meant reduced stigma associated with infections, or at the very least short-lived stigma when considering the 'super-spreader' identities. Yet again, the early moments of COVID-19 saw narratives that seemed to suggest that because only specific groups were susceptible, the need to make collective public health interventions was not urgent, until a recognition of the indiscriminate nature of the pandemic became irrefutable.

Comparisons of HIV/AIDS and SARS-CoV-2/COVID-19 risk destroying efforts and narratives that had been struggled over and built-up to support more complex understandings. Additionally, the power to shape societal viewpoints and the creation of new stories out of remnants after rupture, rests in particularly positioned individuals and institutions, power and privilege entangled in the determination of which narratives are given voice. It may be productive to consider, rather than these two separate pandemics, how forms of power, marginality and public health policy and practice have historically engendered certain narratives, practices and responses that shape different communities' experiences of disease. The different experiences and responses to the pandemics can be argued to reveal more about the structures and relations of our societies and hegemonic narratives of health, disease and illness, than about the viruses or diseases themselves. Though the North American and Western European contexts cannot be used as a universal representation, they offer instructive insights into why comparison here is not inherently useful, or how it can be done productively.

**Florian Zitzelsberger:** My contributions to this roundtable discussion are concerned with the staged presence of AIDS as well as its remediation under the precept of social distancing in the US today. I maintain that there is great promise in how this presence can form a foundation for solidarity, pass criticism on society, or point toward more livable futures, both discursively and materially. We see this perhaps most prominently in how both online and offline performances continue to contribute to support organizations like the Actors Fund or Broadway Cares (visitors of Broadway will likely have encountered their 'red buckets' at some point) or even institutions like amfAR. However, these examples do not effectively compare AIDS and COVID-19. I similarly refrain from making a clear comparison of the two pandemics even though we can witness similar strategies when it comes to marking the virus—and by extension those affected by it—as foreign, as Other. It is important to note that this framing is not meant to homogenize pandemic experiences across time, nor can it adequately describe the differences that arise from the ways both viruses spread, which eventually takes over and shapes their respective narratives. I thus emphatically agree with Dickel's remarks on the role of shame in discourses surrounding AIDS as it pertains to the association of HIV with sexual transmission against the backdrop of homophobia and stigmatization.

I would not necessarily argue that the performed presence of AIDS during COVID-19 aims to straddle this divide to make the *comparison* of the two pandemics productive. On the contrary, these performances do not use AIDS to give solutions for or point to ways of dealing with the COVID-19 pandemic. What they do, however, is bring AIDS back into the consciousness of their audiences. While some of the examples discussed, such as the lockdown performances, directly relate to the COVID-19 pandemic in that they re-envision performance when the co-presence in the theater is not possible, the plays they reference do not. *Angels in America* and *Falsettos*, as well as *The Book of Mormon* and *A Strange Loop*, which I discuss below, were all written and premiered before the COVID-19 pandemic, with the former two constituting contemporary responses to HIV/AIDS of the 1980s and 1990s.

It is my contention that these performances make the *differences* between the two pandemics productive: By not addressing directly the context in which audiences may witness them, the examples discussed force those attending or viewing to decide for themselves how what they see relates to their own experiences and what impact it may have on their lives during the COVID-19 pandemic. Melanie Kreitler (2023) conceptualizes this potential of separate experiences to enrich each other via the *experiential gap*: Applied to my examples, we can thus acknowledge that AIDS and COVID-19 as well as their attendant pandemic experiences are necessarily different while also understanding how the representation of the former can impact on actual experiences of individuals confronted with the latter. The gap Kreitler refers to thus becomes a contact zone rather than an insurmountable divide; it does not result in a collapse of distinct perspectives. In this context, Masamha and Mhishi's comment regarding the underlying structures—power, marginalization, hegemonic narratives of disease and othering—such responses point to seems particularly important. It is not the purpose of AIDS drama to speak to the underlying structures that shape the way individuals experience othering during COVID-19. However, they allow us to find purpose in the (narrative) ruptures between the pandemics—to mind the gap as we find our own ways to move forward.

## How do other factors of social differentiation – beyond those already discussed – intersect with and complicate narratives of disease?

**Roselyne Masamha and Lennon Mhishi:** Migrancy, race and African identity as intersecting factors of social differentiation, provide an important lens through which disease discourses can be analyzed and understood. In particular, 'racialized disease othering,' with recognition of how the kinds of othering accompanying the SARS-CoV-2/COVID-19 pandemic, function in similar and racialized ways (Anti-Asian) as the anti-Black, especially African tropes around Human Immunodeficiency Virus (HIV) and Acquired Immunodeficiency Syndrome (AIDS) as racialized and stigmatized conditions.

Racialization of disease posits one group as 'carriers and purveyors of disease' against another group as 'victims' of the diseased Other. The construction of Africa and Africans as vectors of pathogens, as polluted and polluting, finds early expression in the experiences of slavery and colonialism. This understanding of Africans and Blackness as coterminous with pathogenic life serves not just the function of unhumaning/dehumanization, but also shapes the structures of science and knowledge, and consequently biomedical and biopolitical interventions. In this space, and amongst these people, who exist on these terms outside 'civilizational' time, the strangest and most harmful pathogens abound. From travelogue to missionary narrative and the colonial record, the intersections of race, mobility and disease are present.

It is against such a historical background that the deleterious impacts of HIV/AIDS (and also Ebola) and now SARS-CoV-2/COVID-19 can be read. It is not, as has been apparent, the virus that has any inherent racial character. Rather, the social conditions within which it becomes a disease, and the manner of the response to this, concerns us. These socio-economic and political conditions, existing at a planetary scale yet experienced in very localized ways, (re)produce these forms of racialization of disease, and the stigma and othering that accompany them. The historically produced conditions of stigma and othering, themselves part of larger health disparities, have also been part of the regimes of regulating mobilities and the representations of such mobilities. Migration—as a discourse—has always been at the center of the UK HIV/AIDS epidemic, for example.

The infrastructures of bordering and surveillance intensified as part of efforts to mitigate the impacts of the pandemic, have already existed as part of the intimate lives of migrants. Navigating the institutional and everyday aspects of these infrastructures, subject to various forms of monitoring and limitations in their day-to-day life, migrants have found themselves confronting the border in more severe ways—doubly locked down. Thus, the co-existing identities of migrant-diseased Other coalesce to shape perceptions of, and responses to health and medical institutions, resulting in mistrust, distance and what, in the context of COVID-19, has been characterized as hesitancy by minoritized communities.

COVID-19 and its aftermath magnify the vulnerability of marginalized groups who through deep-seated social and economic inequalities are not only at greater risk of infection, but further disproportionately affected by containment measures and their socioeconomic consequences. The bordering regimes continue to function in ways that entrench pre-existing hierarchies—for instance; announcements that those vaccinated in Africa, Asia and South America would still be considered unvaccinated when they travel to the UK; the selective red-listing of countries; doubly locked down migrants' vulnerabilities to COVID-19 in detention centers and subsequent deportations demonstrating how the borders were 'open' for deportation, yet not for entry.

What then can we learn from the histories of experiences of and responses to HIV/AIDS, from the Global South? Not just as geography and place, but as a set of ideas, practices and imaginaries, and a locus of enacting forms of care and solidarity, as well as understanding, integral to an equitable and just response to pandemics? In other terms, what are the corollaries of this learning for an 'aftermath' in the making, in which claims to building back better may not be accompanied by the actual actions to ensure that, in the face of glaring health disparities. Additionally, where the desperately sought after 'return to normal' translates into a return to the same unfavorable conditions for marginalized groups.

**Florian Zitzelsberger:** When visiting the United States in 2022, for the first time since the start of the COVID-19 pandemic, I was reminded of how mobility figures as a precondition of the pandemic situation we are experiencing and how mobility has always played a major role in this regard. While othering often happens at the intersection with migrancy, I believe that it is a different kind of mobility that has greater bearing on the outbreak of a viral pandemic itself, and that mobility comes from a privileged position: From early settlers who brought with them viruses that were not endemic and thus dangerous to Native North American populations to increasing globalization, business trips, and tourism, epidemics and pandemics show how what Sontag describes as the cultural script of plague is a construct used to mask our own complicity in the pandemic. Society holds on to the idea that "the disease invariably comes from somewhere else" (Sontag 2002, 133) in order to have a scapegoat: SARS-CoV-2 becomes the 'China Virus,' HIV the 'gay virus,' and this script has once again been actualized during the 2022 outbreak of monkeypox, at first also identified as stemming from a 'gay virus.'

Among the Broadway shows I saw between March and April were *The Book of Mormon* and *A Strange Loop*, both of which won the Tony Award for best musical. Notably, both deal with AIDS as a racialized discourse, albeit in vastly different ways. Part of this surely has to do with their two different times of production, with *The Book of Mormon* premiering on Broadway in 2011 and *A Strange Loop* in 2022. *The Book of Mormon* reinforces the cultural script of plague by envisioning Mormon missionaries who leave the United States to help Ugandans in their lives plagued by poverty, famine, and AIDS. The Ugandans—the racial Other—appear as a uniform mass rather than individuals; they serve as a projection surface for discourses of disease, which is further supported by stereotypical characterizations that have led to accusations of racism.

*A Strange Loop* is the story of Usher, a black gay writer working as an usher at a musical, who writes a musical about Usher, a black gay writer working as an usher at a musical, who writes, etc. The show focuses on one individual and all other actors take on the role of Usher's Thoughts, which turns the show into a complex self-exploration. AIDS in *A Strange Loop* is not projected onto a different continent, but is consciously placed in the here-and-now of the performance. An intersectional lens allows the show to highlight the complexities of AIDS within a social group rather than severing the self's ties to it by projecting it onto an Other. *A Strange Loop* shows how a group that is already vulnerable to discrimination based on its association with a virus is divided by religious beliefs regarding Black male homosexuality: "as we prepare to bury yet another un-HBO-special, un-Oscar-So-White-award-winning, ab*Normal-Heart*ed, un-*Angel-in-American* Black queer in the ground, it's very important that we remember what Gawd's word, your word, [Tyler Perry's] word, and every fuckin' body else's word tells us: AIDS IS GOD'S PUNISHMENT" (Jackson 2020, 83). In addition to the two shows' different approaches to AIDS resulting from temporal difference, differing genre ascriptions, and/or their distinct casting choices, with the latter featuring only queer BIPOC individuals in its principal cast, Whitfeld points out that *A Strange Loop*'s Usher is "so clearly a response to creator Michael R. Jackson's own identity as a black queer writer" (2020, 9). I argue that it is this connection to the lived experience of Jackson, who not only wrote the book for the show but also composed its score, that results in *A Strange Loop* being more aware of (or perhaps more sensitive towards) the way discourses surrounding AIDS have historically affected (and continue to do so) Black communities, specifically Black queer men.

Neither of the shows allows the audience to keep up a façade of innocence; instead, they point to—and point out—its complicity in discourses of othering: *The Book of Mormon*, as a comedy, makes the audience laugh at the misfortune of its characters and *A Strange Loop* has the audience clap along as Usher's Thoughts (all played by queer BIPOC individuals) preach their anti-AIDS gospel, a disavowal of queer-of-Color experiences. No matter how caricature-like or differentiated their representations of AIDS are, both examples emphasize that in public consciousness some bodies are a priori associated with disease—or regarded as diseased. However, while *The Book of Mormon* draws a rigid connection between AIDS and Africanness or Blackness (and implicitly religious difference), *A Strange Loop* looks to the United States and the discrimination a fat gay Black man faces and how the association with AIDS leads to an othered position at the intersection of Blackness and male homosexuality to foreground the nuances of having to live with the stigma of being Black and queer in the US today—demonstrating that AIDS is no specter of the past.

**Simon Dickel:** Diseases affect human beings, and human beings are positioned along multiple axes of difference that need to be considered when addressing narratives of diseases. Following Roselyne Masamha, Lennon Mhishi, and Florian Zitzelsberger's views on the importance of the category of race, I would like to remind us that from the 1980s onwards, Black gay activists had criticized how the dominant construction of gay identity as white lead to the false and harmful idea that Black persons were not at risk of contracting HIV. This generation of Black gay artists, activists, filmmakers, and writers, such as Essex Hemphill, Joseph Beam, and Marlon Riggs worked tirelessly to change that perception. The two anthologies *Brother to Brother: New Writings by Black Gay Men* (1991), as well as *Sojourner: Black Gay Voices in the Age of AIDS* (1993), collect texts that address HIV/AIDS in light of the intersections of homosexuality and blackness. It is a good thing that this ground-breaking work is now continued and accessible to a much broader audience through plays, such as *A Strange Loop*, and TV-shows, such as *Pose*.

In addition to this view on cultural negotiations of diseases in relation to categories of difference and to Roselyne Masamha and Lennon Mhishi's emphasis on the centrality of socio-economic conditions, a perspective that includes the dimension of the body and lived experience is needed when addressing the consequences of stigmatization. I think we should pay attention to the ways in which racist, anti-queer, or ableist discourses inscribe themselves into the bodies of human beings, because this bodily dimension of stigmatization has very real consequences for the ways human beings are affected by diseases.

## Works Cited

### Simon Dickel

Butler, Judith. 2016. *Frames of War: When Is Life Grievable?* London: Verso.

Dannecker, Martin. 2022. "Die Zeit von Aids." In *Alle Uns: Differenz, Identität, Repräsentation*, edited by Simon Dickel and Rebecca Racine Ramershoven, 326–39. Münster: Edition Assemblage.

Eribon, Didier. (1999) 2004. *Insult and the Making of the Gay Self*. Durham: Duke University Press.

Hemphill, Essex, ed. 1991. *Brother to Brother: New Writings by Black Gay Men*. Boston: Alyson.

Krasny, Elke. 2020. "In-Sorge-Bleiben: Care-Feminismus für einen Infizierten Planeten." In *Die Corona Gesellschaft: Analysen zur Lage und Perspektiven für die Zukunft*, edited by Michael Volkmar and Karin Werner, 405–14. Bielefeld: transcript.

Odets, Walt. 2019. *Out of the Shadows: Reimagining Gay Men's Lives*. New York: Picador.

Other Countries, eds. 1994. *Sojourner: Black Gay Voices in the Age of AIDS*. New York: Other Countries.

### Roselyne Masamha and Lennon Mhishi

Cole, Teju. 2015. "Unmournable Bodies." *The New Yorker: Cultural Comment*. January 9, 2015. https://www.newyorker.com/culture/cultural-comment/unmournable-bodies.

The Foreign Press Association, Africa—FPAA (@FPA_Africa). 2022. "OUR STATEMENT: The Foreign Press Association, Africa registers its displeasure against media outlets using images of black people alongside stories of the #monkeypox outbreak in North America and the United Kingdom."

Twitter, May 21, 2022, 2:32 p.m. https://twitter.com/FPA_Africa/status/15 27990596044001282/photo/1.

Goffman Erving. 1963. *Stigma: Notes on the Management of Spoiled Identity*. New York: Simon & Shuster.

Ihekweazu, Chikwe (@Chikwe_I). 2021. "This headline from @rheinpfalz referring to the Omicron variant as 'The virus out of Africa' is derogatory, simply wrong & harms the public health response. It creates a damaging narrative and negatively impacts attempts at global solidarity. #Solidarity." Twitter, December 5, 2021, 10:52 p.m. https://twitter.com/Chikwe_I/status/146761 2834381156357/photo/1.

Jones, David S. 2020. "History in a Crisis–Lessons for COVID-19." *New England Journal of Medicine* (April). https://doi.org/10.1056/NEJMp2004361.

Roelen, Keetie, Caroline Ackley, Paul Boyce, Nicolas Farina, and Santiago Ripoll. 2020. "COVID-19 in LMICs: The Need to Place Stigma Front and Centre to Its Response." *The European Journal of Development Research* 32: 1592–612. https://doi.org/10.1057/s41287-020-00316-6.

Sontag, Susan. 1978. *Illness As Metaphor*. New York: Farrar, Straus and Giroux.

World Health Organization. 2020. "Social Stigma Associated with COVID-19." February 24, 2020. https://www.who.int/publications/i/item/social-stigm a-associated-with-covid-19.

## Florian Zitzelsberger

Broadwaycom. 2020. "Scenes from ANGELS IN AMERICA in Support of amfAR's Fund to Fight Covid-19." By Tony Kushner, Theater Play, uploaded October 9, 2020. YouTube, https://www.youtube.com/watch?v=g80_jGJV5qw.

Finn, William, and James Lapine. 1995. *Falsettos*. New York: Samuel French.

Grossman, Max. 2020. "Falsettos In Quarantine." Uploaded May 22, 2020. YouTube, https://www.youtube.com/watch?v=H2z0r73qCFs.

Jackson, Michael R. 2020. *A Strange Loop: A Musical*. New York: Theatre Communications Group.

Kreitler, Melanie. Forthcoming 2023. "Immersive Mental Spaces and the Intersectionally Embodied Self: Representing Mental Illness in Complex (Interactive) Films." In *Shifting Perspectives on Intersectionality*, edited by Grit Grigoleit-Richter and Florian Zitzelsberger. Darmstadt: wbg.

Kushner, Tony. 2013. *Angels in America: A Gay Fantasia on National Themes*. Revised Edition. New York: Theatre Communications Group.

Parker, Trey, Robert Lopez, and Matt Stone. 2011. *The Book of Mormon*. New York: Harper Collins.

Shotwell, Alexis. 2014. "'Women Don't Get AIDS, They Just Die from It': Memory, Classification, and the Campaign to Change the Definition of AIDS." *Hypatia* 29, no. 2: 509–25.

Sontag, Susan. 2002. *Illness as Metaphor & AIDS and Its Metaphors*. London: Penguin.

Waterman, Bryan. 2020. "Plague Time (Again)." *American Literature* 92, no. 4: 759–66.

Whitfeld, Sarah K. 2020. "Disrupting Heteronormative Temporality through Queer Dramaturgies: Fun Home, Hadestown and A Strange Loop." *Arts* 9, no. 69: 1–13.

Zitzelsberger, Florian. 2022. "Presenting AIDS: COVID-19 and the Aesthetics of Social Distance." *Amerikastudien/American Studies* 67, no. 4: 475–88.

# Authors

Simon Dickel, Dr., is Professor of Gender and Diversity Studies at Folkwang University of the Arts in Essen, Germany. Among his recent publications are the book *Embodying Difference: Critical Phenomenology and Narratives of Disability, Race, and Sexuality* (Palgrave Macmillan, 2022) and the co-edited volumes *Alle Uns: Differenz, Identität, Repräsentation* (edition assemblage, 2022) and *Queer Cinema* (Ventil, 2018). His short film *Ready for Ransom* was selected for the 39th Kasseler Dokfest (2022) and the German Competition of the 39th Kurzfilm Festival Hamburg (2023).

Julia Eckel, Dr., is Junior Professor for Film Studies at the Department of Media Studies at Paderborn University, Germany. She is currently working on a book on the nexus of animation, documentation, and demonstration and is also interested in animation and AI, audiovisual anthropomorphism, tech-demos, synthespians, screencasting, and selfies. Recent publications include: *Das Audioviduum. Eine Theoriegeschichte des Menschenmotivs in audiovisuellen Medien* (transcript, 2021) and the co-edited volume *Exploring the Selfie – Historical, Theoretical, and Analytical Approaches to Digital Self-Photography* (Palgrave Macmilan, 2018; with J. Ruchatz and S. Wirth).

Martin Gabriel, Dr., holds a doctorate in history from the University of Klagenfurt, Austria, where he has been working as a lecturer in Modern and Austrian History since 2012. His research focuses on global history and the history of empires between the sixteenth and nineteenth century (with special consideration of Spanish rule in the Americas and its ramifications in the fields of social, economic, and medical history).

Claudia Jahnel, Dr., is Professor for World Christianity and Religious Studies at the University of Hamburg, Germany. Her special interest in research is on the colonial and postcolonial entanglements and negotiations of body-related stereotypes and epistemologies.

Elisa Linseisen, Dr., is Junior Professor of digital, audiovisual media at the University of Hamburg. Her research focuses on the episteme of digital media, apps and post-cinema. She got her doctor's degree with a thesis on "High Definition. Media Philosophical Image Processing" in 2019.

Martin Lüthe, Dr., is currently a visiting professor at the John F. Kennedy Institute for North American Studies at Freie Universität Berlin in Germany, former assistant professor, and Einstein Junior Fellow. He published the monographs *"We Missed a Lot of Church, So the Music Is Our Confessional": Rap and Religion* (Lit Verlag, 2008) and *Color-Line and Crossing-Over: Motown and Performances of Blackness in 1960s American Culture* (WVT, 2011). He also co-edited a volume on *Unpopular Culture* (Amsterdam UP, 2016; with Sascha Pöhlmann) and is on the editorial board of *Eludamos: Journal for Computer Game Culture*.

Roselyne Masamha, Dr., is an independent researcher and clinical educator with a clinical practice background in forensic learning disability nursing. Her research interests and publications are interdisciplinary, spanning across mental health nursing, clinical supervision, the experiences of marginalized groups, migration, feminist critical thought and decolonial tensions.

Lennon Mhishi, Dr., is a researcher at the University of Oxford's Pitt Rivers Museum, United Kingdom, working at the intersections of colonial collections, restitution, contemporary art practice and epistemic plurality. His interdisciplinary work spans interests in the afterlives of slavery and colonialism, the African diaspora, mobility and displacement, music and belonging, and recently, creative heritage and community-based approaches to forms of exploitation, forced labor and human rights in different African countries. He is particularly interested in film, music, sound and other arts-based, creative approaches to knowledge-making and engagement.

Natalie Pielok is a PhD candidate in Media Studies at the Ruhr University Bochum, Germany. In addition to her curatorial and artistic work, her thematic focus is on media and sound theory, gender, queer and postcolonial studies. She has been working for Professor Dr. Henriette Gunkel's professorship of "Transformations of Audiovisual Media with a Special Focus on Gender and Queer Theory" since 2020.

Romana Radlwimmer, Dr., is Professor for Romance Literatures (with a special focus on Hispanophone and Lusophone Literatures) at the Goethe University of Frankfurt, Germany. She is the director of two VW-funded projects *Pandemics and Coloniality: Biopolitical Entanglements in Early Modern Chronicles and COVID-19 Narratives*, and *Archives of Colonial Dis/Possesion: Centering Non-European Perspectives on Wealth (15th–18th Centuries)*. Her research interests include contemporary Latin American literatures and theories, urban literatures of the Iberian Peninsula, and sixteenth to seventeenth century Spanish and Portuguese Colonial Literature.

Anke Scherer, Dr., is an Assistant Professor of Japanese History at Ruhr-University Bochum's Faculty of East Asian Studies in Germany. Her research interests include cultural narratives and Japanese imperialism, particularly in Manchuria and Taiwan. Her current research focus is on public hygiene in imperial Japan.

Heike Steinhoff, Dr., is Junior Professor of American Studies at Ruhr-University Bochum, Germany. She is the author of *Transforming Bodies: Makeovers and Monstrosities in American Culture* (Palgrave Macmillan, 2015) and *Queer Buccaneers: (De)Constructing Boundaries in the Pirates of the Caribbean Film Series* (Lit, 2011). Among her recent publications is also the edited volume *Hipster Culture: Transnational and Intersectional Perspectives* (Bloomsbury, 2021). Her research focuses on American media culture, gender studies, urban studies, and intersectional feminist studies of the human body.

Martin Tschiggerl, Dr., is a historian and completed his PhD in Vienna, Austria in 2018 with a thesis on the construction of national identity and alterity in the three successor societies of the Nazi state. After working in Berlin, Chicago and Saarbrücken, he has been a research associate at the Institute for Cultural Studies of the Austrian Academy of Sciences since 2022. His research focuses on contemporary and cultural history, theory of science and media, as well as digital and public history.

Danielle Heberle Viegas, Dr., is a Brazilian historian of cities, with an emphasis on urban planning and the environment. She holds a PhD in Ibero-American History from PUCRS Brazil and Freie Universität Berlin (2016). After concluding her professorship at Universidade La Salle in Canoas (2020), she joined the Munich Centre for Global History to attend the special program *Corona Crisis and Beyond* funded by Volkswagen Stiftung (2021). Following her post-doctoral research at LMU München in Germany, she became the P.I. of the Gerda Henkel project *Resilient Forest Cities: Utopia and Development in the Brazilian Amazon*, hosted at the Max-Planck Institute of Geoanthropology (2023–2026).

Florian Zitzelsberger is a PhD candidate in American Studies at the University of Passau, Germany, whose research is situated at the intersections of queer theory, performance studies, and narrative theory. Among others, his work has appeared in *Amerikastudien*, *Humanities*, and the *Journal of Narrative Theory*. He is co-editor of "Posthuman Drag," a special issue of *Queer Studies in Media & Popular Culture*.

# [transcript]

# PUBLISHING.
# KNOWLEDGE. TOGETHER.

transcript publishing stands for a multilingual transdisciplinary pro-gramme in the social sciences and humanities. Showcasing the latest academic research in various fields and providing cutting-edge diagno-ses on current affairs and future perspectives, we pride ourselves in the promotion of modern educational media beyond traditional print and e-publishing. We facilitate digital and open publication formats that can be tailored to the specific needs of our publication partners.

## OUR SERVICES INCLUDE

- partnership-based publishing models
- Open Access publishing
- innovative digital formats: HTML, Living Handbooks, and more
- sustainable digital publishing with XML
- digital educational media
- diverse social media linking of all our publications

Visit us online: www.transcript-publishing.com

Find our latest catalogue at www.transcript-publishing.com/newbookspdf

GPSR Authorized Representative: Easy Access System Europe, Mustamäe tee
50, 10621 Tallinn, Estonia, gpsr.requests@easproject.com

www.ingramcontent.com/pod-product-compliance
Lightning Source LLC
Chambersburg PA
CBHW061728120626
46550CB00005B/1741